Trauma and Trauma Consequence Disorder

Markus J. Pausch · Sven J. Matten

Trauma and Trauma Consequence Disorder

In Media, Management and Public

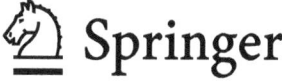

Markus J. Pausch
Munich, Germany

Sven J. Matten
Munich, Germany

ISBN 978-3-658-38806-5   ISBN 978-3-658-38807-2 (eBook)
https://doi.org/10.1007/978-3-658-38807-2

© The Editor(s) (if applicable) and The Author(s), under exclusive license to Springer Fachmedien Wiesbaden GmbH, part of Springer Nature 2022
This work is subject to copyright. All rights are solely and exclusively licensed by the Publisher, whether the whole or part of the material is concerned, specifically the rights of translation, reprinting, reuse of illustrations, recitation, broadcasting, reproduction on microfilms or in any other physical way, and transmission or information storage and retrieval, electronic adaptation, computer software, or by similar or dissimilar methodology now known or hereafter developed.
The use of general descriptive names, registered names, trademarks, service marks, etc. in this publication does not imply, even in the absence of a specific statement, that such names are exempt from the relevant protective laws and regulations and therefore free for general use.
The publisher, the authors, and the editors are safe to assume that the advice and information in this book are believed to be true and accurate at the date of publication. Neither the publisher nor the authors or the editors give a warranty, expressed or implied, with respect to the material contained herein or for any errors or omissions that may have been made. The publisher remains neutral with regard to jurisdictional claims in published maps and institutional affiliations.

Responsible Editor: Eva Brechtel-Wahl
This Springer imprint is published by the registered company Springer Fachmedien Wiesbaden GmbH, part of Springer Nature.
The registered company address is: Abraham-Lincoln-Str. 46, 65189 Wiesbaden, Germany

Foreword by Till Krauseneck

Why a book on trauma and trauma-related disorders in the media, management and the public?

In my opinion, there are at least three good reasons:

1. The risk of being exposed to particularly severe events and experiences is at least as high for people in this field of work as for any other people. The use of help may be impeded by the existing implicit aura of being able to function and perform even under high pressure. There is also the loneliness of being left to oneself—both in terms of decisions and burdens—and the fact that this can be expressed less, which adds to the problem. To make the severe suffering caused by trauma and the sometimes serious restrictions on life, which have so far remained hidden under the smooth surface of professionalism, accessible, this book—discreetly in self-study—can provide knowledge to those affected, show the way to treatment and/or give concrete suggestions for self-help.
2. Not only in everyday life but also in professional settings such as clinical practice, the correct symptom classification and the correct diagnosis are still not carried out continuously and often with delay. This is partly due to the diverse symptomatology. On the other hand, despite the constant increase in knowledge and the now existing variety of methods, the importance and significance of trauma are still underestimated not only for PTSD but also for the genesis, maintenance and treatment of many other mental disorders.

    In many affective disorders, addictions, personality disorders and anxiety and obsessive-compulsive disorders, past traumas often represent a significant influencing factor and have a great influence on the course and treatment.

    In order to prevent an inflationary use and an improper simplification or attribution of causality and to correctly classify comorbidities, this book offers a good orientation. The clear, systematic—including the integrated current classifications—and structured, focused on the essentials and at the same time comprehensive representation including the concrete and tried and tested techniques and treatment suggestions in a clear scope are a good starting point and faithful companion for those active in the medical field.
3. The greatest strength of this well-written and fluid book is that it builds a bridge and makes the often difficult to convey symptomatology comprehensible and comprehensible or, in the best sense, comprehensible. This is mainly due to the particularly well-formulated and concise case examples in which the cooperation and the different perspectives of a specialized therapist and a media manager become experience-readable and readable. The current evidence-based state of knowledge is overviewed across schools and reflected in a very understandable way for laymen. This is particularly important because the comparison of the individual symptoms and experiences with the existing classification and terminology is essential for both diagnosis and recognition of the underlying problems and treatment.

A model of explanation developed and worked out together by those affected and treated, illustrated and plausible, forms the foundation of a common language that is indispensable for coping with the symptomatology and regaining control.

Till Krauseneck
Head of Department of Psychosomatics,
Psychiatry and Psychotherapy at
kbo-Isar-Amper-Klinikum Munich-Ost

Foreword by Karin Parkhof

The two authors have succeeded in writing a reference book on trauma and trauma sequelae that is aimed at many readers, especially those who are in the public eye, hold a leadership position or come from this environment, and not only, as is usually the case, at therapists.

The many and good case examples illustrate the symptoms of trauma and trauma sequelae in an impressive and comprehensible way. The book gives affectedaffected persons help for self-help and supports the people who work with an affected person in their immediate environment or live together with them in a partnership.

Even managers can benefit from this book. In companies, more and more people are working who are directly or indirectly affectedaffected by burnout, anxiety disorders, trauma or post-traumatic stress disorder, and who also come from other cultures, such as Syria or Afghanistan. Management then faces the question: Why are these people so different? What have they experienced? Are these the cultural differences or am I taking symptoms of a possible post-traumatic stress disorder? How do I lead these people? Who can advise and support me? Here the book provides valuable information.

People working in public relations can also gain important impulses for their work. Whoever writes about people—sometimes writes about destinies. Maybe an interesting story that boosts sales figures—but it is also the story of a person or of many people who may have to suffer from the events for a lifetime. I would like to see a responsible, sensitive approach and a careful weighing up, taking into account the interests of the person concerned. This book is an invitation to do so.

This book has made me more aware of how I treat my colleagues at Siemens. It encouraged me to act accordingly in my role as organizer of seminars on work and leadership techniques, cooperation and health, to break the silence, to make conversation offers—if they are desired. I realized that it is not about individual destinies, but that many more people are affectedaffected than I had assumed.

"Trauma and Post-Traumatic Stress Disorder—In the Media, Management and Public"
A professional book for people who want to deal with the topic in more depth, for those directly and indirectly affected, especially in exposed positions, as well as for laypeople. A book that explains, supports and encourages.

Looking away has never helped—looking is one facet of humanity.

Karin Parkhof
Siemens AG

Contents

1	**Introduction**	1
2	**Trauma and Posttraumatic Stress Disorder (PTSD)—Definition, Classification, Epidemiology and History**	3
2.1	What is a Trauma?—Trauma Definition	4
2.2	What Traumas are There?—Classifications of Traumas	5
2.3	Posttraumatic Stress Disorder (PTSD)	6
2.4	Trauma-Related Disorders in Different Classifications	7
2.5	What is How Often?—Epidemiology of PTSD	10
2.6	The History of PTSD as a Diagnosis	11
	References	12
3	**Physiology of a Traumatic Situation**	13
3.1	Why Feelings?—Basics of Emotions	14
3.2	Acute Traumatisation and the Traumatic Pincer	16
3.3	The Unbearable can be Borne!—Dissociation in the Traumatic Situation	19
3.4	Early Intervention and Debriefing—Does Quick Help Help Quickly?	20
3.5	What Protects?—Resilience	23
3.6	What is at Risk?—Risk Factors for PTSD	25
	References	26
4	**Symptoms of PTSD**	27
4.1	Core Symptoms of PTSD	28
4.1.1	Intrusions	29
4.1.2	Hyperarousal	31
4.1.3	Avoidance Behavior	32
4.2	Symptoms of Complex PTSD	34
4.3	Dissociation and Dissociative Identity Structure as a Result of Severe, Complex and Chronic Traumatization	36
4.4	If Something Else Happens!—Comorbidities	39
4.4.1	Anxiety Disorders	40
4.4.2	Depressions	44
4.4.3	Dependency Disorders	45
4.4.4	Other Mental Illnesses	48
4.4.5	Somatic Comorbidities	48
4.5	Self-Injury and Suicidal Thoughts	50
	References	51
5	**Dealing with Trauma and PTSD Privately and in Public**	53
5.1	Am I or the Others Going Crazy?—The Question of the What and Why	54
5.2	Am I to Blame?—The Question of Why	55
5.3	Break the Silence?	56

6	**Trauma Coping and Professional Services**	59
6.1	What Can I Do Myself—Strategies for "Self-Therapeutic" Help	61
6.1.1	If the Memory Keeps Coming Back!—Dealing with Flashbacks, Nightmares, Traumatic Memories	61
6.1.2	Not the Same Thing Again!—Dealing with Avoidance Behavior	65
6.1.3	Always under Pressure!—Dealing with Hyperarousal	67
6.1.4	When Half the Day is Missing!—Dealing with Dissociations	72
6.1.5	When the Mind Falls into the Trap!—The 10 Most Important Cognitive PTSD Traps	74
6.1.6	Thought Carousel!—Dealing with Thought Circles	77
6.1.7	When Fears Determine Life!—Dealing with Fears	78
6.1.8	What to Do about Pain?	79
6.1.9	When the Night Becomes Day!—Dealing with Sleep Disorders	80
6.1.10	When Addiction has You in its Grip!—Dealing with Addiction	81
6.2	**Resources**	81
6.3	**General Basics of Trauma Therapy**	82
6.4	**Behavioral, Psychodynamic and Trauma-Specific Approaches**	84
6.4.1	Stabilization Phase	85
6.4.2	Confrontation Phase	89
6.4.3	Reorientation Phase	89
6.5	**Confrontation Procedures**	90
6.5.1	EMDR	90
6.5.2	Narrative Exposure Therapy (NET)	91
6.5.3	PITT and Observer Technique	91
6.5.4	IRRT	93
6.6	**Medication**	93
	References	94
7	**How the Social Environment of Those Affected by Trauma and PTSD Deals with the Topic**	95
8	**Disease Prevention and Primary/Secondary Traumatization**	99
8.1	**Prevention**	100
8.2	**Secondary Traumatization**	101
	References	101
9	**Trauma and PTSD in Film and Literature**	103
9.1	**Movies with the Theme of Trauma and PTSD**	104
9.2	**Literary Works with the Theme of Trauma and PTSD**	106
10	**Future Prospects, Manage Business and Everyday Life**	109
10.1	**What Can I Do?**	110
10.2	**Understanding as the First Step to a Solution**	111

Supplementary Information

Recommended Reading	114
Index	115

About the Authors

Sven J. Matten MBA
After specializing in the fields of media marketing and direct marketing at the Bavarian Academy of Advertising and Marketing (BAW) in Munich, the Master of Business Administration (MBA) at the European University in Montreux (Switzerland), the Professional Producers Program at the School of Theater, Film and Television at the University of Los Angeles (UCLA) in the USA and the admission to the practice of naturopathy restricted to the field of psychotherapy in Bavaria, Sven J. Matten founded the film production and financing companies Paradigma Entertainment in Munich and DuMatt Entertainment in Winnipeg (Manitoba, Canada), taught at the Munich Business School in the fields of marketing and international media business and today coaches selected personalities in international management and in particularly exposed positions at the locations Munich and Toronto (Ontario, Canada) within the framework of the "phocamento" platform. Specialized in anxiety disorders, Sven J. Matten today coaches selected personalities in international management and in particularly exposed positions at the locations Munich and Toronto (Ontario, Canada).
Sven J. Matten on Wikipedia: ▶ https://de.wikipedia.org/wiki/Sven_J._Matten
Sven J. Matten on LinkedIn: ▶ www.linkedin.com/in/svenjmatten
Write to the author: sjm@phocamento.com

Dr. Markus J. Pausch
After completing his studies in medicine, he first worked as a doctor at the University Hospital of Regensburg in the field of internal medicine. In 2008 he moved from Regensburg to Munich to the kbo-Isar-Amper-Klinikum München Ost. There he completed his training as a specialist in psychiatry and psychotherapy with a focus on geriatric psychiatry, general psychiatry, crisis intervention and addiction medicine. He then worked for one year in the field of neuropsychology. Since 2010 he has been intensively trained in the field of psychotherapy with a focus on psychotraumatology (incl. acute traumatization), early disorders and consequences / comorbidities of a mental traumatization (focus on anxiety disorders). Since 2017 he has been an EMDRIA certified EMDR therapist and senior physician of the trauma center at the kbo-Isar-Amper-Klinikum München.
Markus J. Pausch on LinkedIn: ▶ www.linkedin.com/in/markusjpausch

Introduction

© The Author(s), under exclusive license to Springer Fachmedien Wiesbaden GmbH, part of Springer Nature 2022
M. J. Pausch and S. J. Matten, *Trauma and Trauma Consequence Disorder*,
https://doi.org/10.1007/978-3-658-38807-2_1

You suddenly have sleep disorders with stressful nightmares, experience a traumatic event over and over again, see images, get strong fears associated with unusual physical symptoms.

You have a flashback in a board meeting or in the checkout line at the supermarket.

You suddenly have a dissociation in the spotlight on a stage or in a train. You suddenly lack half a day.

You are unusually startled in everyday life. Your need to wash suddenly becomes burdensome and compulsive.

You avoid any memories and potentially threatening situations out of fear of re-experiencing.

Traumatic and existential threatening situations happen suddenly and affect many people. But only a part of them develop post-traumatic stress disorder (PTSD).

What protects the one from it and how can the affected person deal with the symptoms independently? Why is he affected and why not?

What makes a trauma a trauma, what are the symptoms of post-traumatic stress disorder at all? And is it a weakness to have such symptoms? Maybe even a strength?

How can one deal constructively with traumas and post-traumatic stress disorders, especially in exposed positions? Use and overcome these perhaps even as a competitive advantage, regain personal happiness?

Does this only concern me, or are there others as well? And how do I deal with a person who has experienced a trauma?

By the combined look of an experienced psychiatric medical therapist and a long-time manager, this book is the fusion of a practice-oriented textbook with a professional guide. Interrelationships and solutions for coping with trauma, especially for exposed persons, are shown. Self-initiative and a possible need for professional support are expressly not replaced. The aim is to gain knowledge.

Sometimes the female, sometimes the male form is used below. Of course, unless otherwise stated, all genders are meant to be equal. For reasons of efficiency, given the target group of media/management/public, only the most essential information is focused on and thus dispenses with detailed descriptions and background information. An extensive bibliography serves as a guide for deepening individual interests. The index helps the reader to quickly find specific information, sorted by keywords.

Trauma and management, fear and public, and also all connecting media—all these aspects are closely related. Often it is precisely such inner drives as traumatic experiences and their consequences that make people particularly successful in management and public. But knowledge, understanding and the right approach are decisive. This also applies to the optimal use of one's own resources, both in terms of professional career and in the simultaneous pursuit of personal happiness. It is important and unavoidable to accept what has happened radically and to use it actively to your advantage. This means not closing your eyes, accepting the challenge and growing from it. Not easy at all, but is there really any alternative?

Trauma and Posttraumatic Stress Disorder (PTSD)—Definition, Classification, Epidemiology and History

Contents

2.1 What is a Trauma?—Trauma Definition – 4

2.2 What Traumas are There?—Classifications of Traumas – 5

2.3 Posttraumatic Stress Disorder (PTSD) – 6

2.4 Trauma-Related Disorders in Different Classifications – 7

2.5 What is How Often?—Epidemiology of PTSD – 10

2.6 The History of PTSD as a Diagnosis – 11

References – 12

© The Author(s), under exclusive license to Springer Fachmedien Wiesbaden GmbH, part of Springer Nature 2022
M. J. Pausch and S. J. Matten, *Trauma and Trauma Consequence Disorder*,
https://doi.org/10.1007/978-3-658-38807-2_2

Traumatic events have been part of his life since there have been humans. At all times, man has also been confronted with the apparently unbearable, the existentially threatening and the power and violence of nature and fellow human beings in his being. In some professions, humans are more exposed to such risks than in others. Events that are experienced as traumatic are characterized by the fact that they trigger psychological, cognitive, physical and emotional stress in the affected person. The feeling of helplessness, of being overwhelmed, of powerlessness can arise. But it can also be that a person does not feel anything at all in a traumatic situation. Many different reactions are conceivable, possible and normal. Traumatizations that take place to a large extent and early in a person's life often have far-reaching and deep effects on the affected person.

2.1 What is a Trauma?—Trauma Definition

There is no universally valid definition of mental trauma (Greek for "wound"). The term has changed over the past years and decades. A basic idea was and is that, like a physical trauma, it is an injury. A trauma injures the human soul and leads to a wound.

In 1991, the World Health Organization (WHO) defined a trauma as "a short- or long-term event or occurrence of extraordinary threat with catastrophic dimensions that would cause deep despair in almost everyone."

A traumatic situation is characterized by a **discrepancy** between the **subjectively experienced threat to oneself or others** and the **individual coping strategies**. So it is not necessary that the affected persons see the danger to life for themselves. It can also be traumatizing for someone if the danger to life for others is feared, e.g. when observing violence. In addition, the sudden loss of a important reference person or a life-threatening illness can lead to an overload of the individual coping strategies.

Traumas are events that can be characterized by their **suddenness** ("It happens out of the blue."), their **severity** ("There are destructive forces at work with the danger to health and life."), and their **hopelessness** ("One is helpless and exposed.").

Often an attempt is made to make a trauma tangible by saying that such an event would throw every person more or less off course.

A sentence that affected people often say is the following: **"After that, nothing was like it was before!"**

This sentence is very accurate. But it also implies that there was a "before". Not infrequently, the traumatization began so early in life that the affected person can no longer remember such a "before".

In the event of trauma, those affected experience physical, cognitive and emotional reactions. On the physical level, a massive stress reaction occurs. This manifests itself, among other things, in heart palpitations, increased blood pressure, sweating, trembling, dizziness, nausea. On the cognitive level, the only possible thought is often that one is about to die. In some cases, there is also partial amnesia for the phase of traumatization, which leads to the fact that the affected persons have only limited memories of the event. Emotionally, a reaction can occur during traumatization, but complete emotional numbness can also occur. In the latter case, the affected persons experience the traumatic situation without feeling anything.

There is emotional silence in the affected persons. If an emotional reaction occurs, it is characterized by fear, anxiety, panic, helplessness, hopelessness, vulnerability and often a fear of death.

It is important that those affected are made aware that every reaction in the traumatic situation is correct. Everyone reacts in such an extreme situation in the way that is possible for him at the time.

The 10th edition of the "International Statistical Classification of Diseases and Related Health Problems", abbreviated ICD-10, valid in Germany, which the WHO defines as a trauma, is **"a short- or long-term event or event of extraordinary threat with catastrophic dimensions, which would trigger deep despair in almost everyone."**

In the United States valid and published by the American Psychiatric Association (APA; American Psychiatric Association) classification system "Diagnostic and Statistical Manual of Mental Disorders" (DSM; Diagnostic and Statistical Manual of Mental Disorders) a trauma is characterized by the **"actual or threatened confrontation with death, serious injury or sexual violence."** It is further distinguished more precisely in what way such a confrontation can take place: namely by "direct experience", "personal witness", "in the immediate family or close friends" or by the "repeated confrontation with aversive details".

2.2 What Traumas are There?—Classifications of Traumas

There are a variety of events that can be classified as traumatic. These include traffic accidents, natural disasters, violent crimes, robberies, rapes, sexual violence, etc. Different classifications of these many different traumas have been established.

The first division separates the traumatic events according to whether they have occurred once or several times.
- **Type-I-Traumata**: These are events that are characterized by a single trauma. These traumas are usually short-term.
- Examples: car accident, bank robbery
- **Type-II-Traumata**: These include those traumas in which there are several traumatic events. The traumatization is long-term here.
- Examples: sexual abuse, violence experiences over a long period of time

A second, important subdivision separates the events according to the causing instance.
- **Non-intentional/accidental traumas**: These include all those traumatic events that occur randomly and/or are caused by nature.
- Examples: traffic accidents, earthquakes
- **Intentional traumas**: Traumatization caused by people deliberately and intentionally falls into this category. For such traumatization, the terms **man-made-disaster** or **relationship traumatization** have also been established.

It has been shown that the human psyche can better process traumatic events that occur randomly and are caused by nature than those that occur as part of a relationship traumatization. This also seems very plausible, since all interpersonal areas as well as the self-, human- and world image of the victim play a major role in traumatization caused by another person. And in these areas, such traumatization often leads to a change or damage.

Another division can take place according to the age in which the traumatic event occurs. Traumas that occur in early phases of life often fall into phases of special vulnerability in which the personality of the affected person is not yet fully developed. Traumatization in such phases often leaves deeper consequences for the mental health.

2.3 Posttraumatic Stress Disorder (PTSD)

> **PTSD**
>
> The term PTSD is an acronym and results from the initial letters of the term Post-Traumatic Stress-Disorder. The term can be explained as follows: After (ie "post") the experience of a trauma, there is a reaction of stress, that is, a disturbed processing. In Anglo-Saxon and repeatedly in German-speaking countries, the term Post Traumatic Stress Disorder(PTSD) is used.

The fact that a person has experienced one or more traumas does not necessarily mean that the person will develop posttraumatic stress disorder (PTSD).

▶ The principle applies: **"Trauma does not mean PTSD!"**

Often, PTSD is not used as a term, but rather trauma disorder. The term trauma disorder is much broader and includes a much larger range of symptoms, syndromes, disorders and reactions to traumatic events, with the trauma usually not being the sole cause, but rather a risk factor.

Post-traumatic stress disorder is a specific form of trauma disorder. Other forms or related disorders are acute stress reaction, adjustment disorder and ongoing personality change after extreme stress.

Traumatization that is intentional (i.e. caused by a person), happens often and over a long period of time, begins very early in the life of the affected person, involves a very high level of violence or even sexual violence, often leads to a symptomatology that goes beyond that of PTSD. The consequences of such traumatization are usually also a disturbed personality development.

Since the consequences of such complex traumatization are no longer congruent with what is meant by PTSD, the terms "complex trauma disorder" or "complex presentation of PTSD" are often used.

Other trauma disorders include dissociative disorders, somatoform pain disorder, dissociative identity disorder (or better known as dissociative identity structure) and emotionally unstable personality disorder.

In addition, there are some disorders in which the presence of one or more traumas plays an important role in their development. These include eating disorders, affective disorders and dependency disorders.

Post-traumatic stress can, especially if it is chronic, lead to a permanent stress reaction in the body. Such "chronic stress" can contribute to or negatively affect the course of physical diseases. In the current studies on this, this is particularly true for cardiovascular and immunological diseases.

2.4 Trauma-Related Disorders in Different Classifications

In Germany, as in all other European countries, all mental and physical illnesses are classified according to the WHO classification system, the International Statistical Classification of Diseases and Related Health Problems (English: International Statistical Classification of Diseases and Related Health Problems; **ICD**). The current version is the 10th version and is therefore referred to as ICD-10.

Within this classification, is classified as PTBS (ICD-10: F43.1). The ICD-10 provides specific criteria that must be met in order for a diagnosis of PTBS to be made. These diagnostic criteria are as follows:
- "traumatic event of exceptional severity"
- Symptoms appear "within 6 months of" the traumatic event
- "repeated unavoidable memories or re-enactment of the event in memory, daydreams or dreams" (so-called **reliving/intrusions**)
- "avoidance of stimuli that could trigger a memory of the trauma" (so-called **avoidance behavior**) and "emotional numbness" (so-called **numbing**)
- "vegetative disorder" in the form of overexcitability (so-called **hyperarousal/overexcitability**)
- (ICD-10, Dilling et al., 2011)

Reliving, avoidance behavior and overexcitability are the three core symptoms of PTSD.

Often so-called subsyndromal disease patterns are also seen. Here, not all diagnostic criteria for PTSD are met, the disorder is so to speak not fully expressed. Nevertheless, the disorder is PTSD-like.

Other reactions and diagnostic classifications after exposure to severe stress are **acute stress reaction** and **adjustment disorder**.

Diagnostic criteria for **acute stress reaction**:
- "unusual stress"
- Symptoms begin "immediately" or "within minutes" of exposure
- "Mixed and changing picture" with emotional "numbness", "depression, anxiety, anger, despair, hyperactivity and withdrawal", with no one symptom predominating
- Symptoms are "rapidly reversible" and "usually only minimal after 3 days"
- (ICD-10, Dilling et al., 2011)

Acute stress reaction is initially a physiological reaction of the psyche to an extraordinary stress.

Diagnostic criteria for **adjustment disorder**:
- "unusual stress"
- Symptoms begin within one month of the start of the unusual stress

- Different symptoms or changes in social behavior (e.g. aggressive or antisocial behavior) are shown. No symptoms meet the criteria for individual disorders, such as social phobia. Mixed disorders can occur.
- Symptoms last no longer than six months
- (ICD-10, Dilling et al., 2011)

If, in addition to the symptoms of "classic" PTSD, other symptoms occur, it is possible that an additional mental illness is present, e.g. an anxiety disorder. This second disorder may also have developed as a result of a traumatic event.

Those affected who have experienced not one, but several serious traumatic situations, which may have lasted for several years, often show a disorder which includes PTSD (i.e. all diagnostic criteria of PTSD are met), but in its symptomatology goes beyond and has further complaints. This disorder is often referred to as "complex trauma disorder", "complex presentation of PTSD" or "complex PTSD", without any of these terms being universally accepted or there being clear and fixed criteria for this. The term "complex PTSD" was first used by US psychiatrist Judith Herman 1992. There is no diagnostic classification for this form of illness in the ICD-10 and thus no generally accepted criteria for diagnosis.

In his book "Post-traumatic stress disorders" (1998), Andreas Maercker proposed the following diagnostic criteria for complex PTSD:

- **Trauma criterion:** Presence of a long-lasting traumatic event (e.g. victims of organized violence, domestic violence, severe sexual or physical violence in childhood)
- **Core symptoms of PTSD** (re-experiencing, avoidance behavior, numbing, hyperarousal)
- Impairment of additional areas such as
  - Regulation of emotions: Emotions are experienced as unbearable, uncontrollable and there are frequent outbursts of emotion, periods of "numbness", depressive episodes as well as self-injury and thoughts of suicide.
  - Changes in self-image: The affected persons experience themselves as worthless, inferior, bad, guilty and inferior. In addition, there is a feeling of shame.
  - Disruption of relationship formation: Relationships can be difficult to establish due to fear, mistrust, etc., it can be difficult to regulate proximity and distance, and relationships are often abruptly terminated.
  - Occurrence of dissociations.

Another diagnostic classification of complex trauma disorders can be made in the group of ongoing personality disorders after extreme stress in the ICD-10. In the DSM there is no corresponding category. As part of field studies for the DSM-IV, the term and the diagnostic entity of DESNOS ("**D**isorder of **E**xtrem **S**tress **N**ot **O**therwise **S**pecified"; German: Disorder of extreme stress not otherwise specified) were created. However, this diagnosis did not find its way into the classification system DSM in the end. Nevertheless, what is used under this term describes complex trauma very well. For this reason, it is often used in psychiatric, psychotherapeutic everyday life and research.

2.4 · Trauma-Related Disorders in Different Classifications

Diagnostic criteria for **DESNOS** (according to Luxenberg et al., 2001):
- Changes in affect regulation and at least 1 symptom of dealing with anger, self-destructive behavior, suicidality, disturbances of sexuality, excessive risk behavior.
- Amnesia or transient dissociative episodes and depersonalization
- Changes in self-perception with at least 2 symptoms of ineffectiveness, stigmatization, feelings of guilt, shame, isolation, trivialization
- Changes in relationships with others with at least 1 symptom of inability to trust, revictimization, victimization of others
- Somatization with at least 2 symptoms of gastrointestinal symptoms, chronic pain, cardiovascular symptoms, conversion symptoms, sexual symptoms.
- Changes in life attitudes with despair and hopelessness or/and loss of former supporting basic beliefs.
- The earlier in a person's life that traumatization occurs and the longer it lasts, the higher the likelihood that a DESNOS will develop
- (Pelcovitz et al., 1997).

In any case, when there is suspicion of (complex) PTSD and/or other mental illness, a comprehensive diagnostic assessment should be carried out by a qualified professional, preferably with good trauma therapy experience and qualifications.

In the United States of America, mental illnesses are classified according to the Diagnostic and Statistical Manual of Mental Disorders (DSM; German: "Diagnostic and Statistical Manual of Mental Disorders"), published by the American Psychiatric Association (APA). The 5th edition (therefore DSM-5), revised in 2013, was published.

In the previously valid version, DSM-IV, from 1994, the diagnosis of post-traumatic stress disorder was assigned to the anxiety disorders and the following criteria were required:
- experience or observe a traumatic event with potential or actual danger of death, serious injury, threat to physical integrity of oneself or others (so-called **A1 criterion**, or objective characteristic).
- reaction with intense fear, helplessness, horror to this event (so-called **A2 criterion**, or subjective characteristic).
- **re-experiencing** (at least 1 symptom of intrusion, distressing (nightmare) dreams, flashbacks, stress from triggers, physiological reaction to memories).
- **Avoidance** (at least 3 symptoms of avoidance of certain thoughts/feelings, avoidance of certain activities/situations, amnesia, avoidance of certain interests, sense of estrangement, restricted affective range).
- **Excessive arousal** (at least 2 symptoms of insomnia/hypervigilance, increased irritability, concentration difficulties, exaggerated startle response).
- **Time criterion:** duration of the above symptoms for at least 4 weeks.
- (DSM-IV-TR, Saß et al., 1996)

In the new version, the DSM-5 (now with Arabic and no longer Roman numeral) from 2013, there were some small but important changes.

First, PTSD was no longer classified with anxiety disorders, but rather a separate **group for trauma- and stress-related disorders** was created. In this group are now in addition to post-traumatic stress disorder, the acute stress reaction and adjustment disorder. The latter two represent reactions to severe stress, which show different symptoms (e.g. depressive mood, anxiety, flashbacks), but after 1 month (acute stress reaction) or after 6 months (adjustment disorder) disappear again.

Secondly, the A2 criterion, that is, the subjective reaction with intense fear, helplessness or horror to the traumatic event, was given up. With this decision, the American Psychiatric Association, as the publisher of the DSM-5, has adapted the diagnostic criteria of PTSD to a large extent to the reality of those affected. Very often, the traumatic situation is so overwhelming that there is no emotional reaction due to this clear overload. The psyche of those affected is so overwhelmed that the potentially experienced emotions would be unbearable and thus any emotion is "switched off". One could say that the "non-feeling" as a reaction is an intensification of the intense fear, helplessness or horror.

Unfortunately, no separate diagnosis for complex post-traumatic stress disorder was created in the DSM-5. The hopes for such a diagnosis now lie with the new version of the ICD, which is expected to be adopted by the WHO in 2018.

2.5 What is How Often?—Epidemiology of PTSD

The probability that one will become a victim of traumatization in Germany is not as low as one might suspect. Between a quarter and a third of all people living in Germany experience at least one trauma during their lifetime (Maercker et al., 1998). In the United States, the number is much higher, with about 60% of all people experiencing at least one trauma during their lifetime. Of these 60%, only about 8% of men and 20% of women suffer from PTSD (Kessler et al., 1995).

According to a study by Kessler et al. from the year 1995 9.2% of the 5877 subjects were women and 0.7% were men who were victims of rape. Of these, 45% of the women and 65% of the men showed the picture of PTSD. Furthermore, 12.3% (women), or 2.8% (men) experienced sexual abuse in childhood. Of these, 26.5% (women), or 12.2% (men) developed PTSD. Likewise, those who experienced neglect in childhood (3.4% of women; 2.1% of men) showed PTSD in 19.7% (women)/23.9% (men). Those who experienced physical violence (11.1% men; 6.9% women) developed PTSD in 1.8% (men), or 21.3% (women). Men and women who experienced violence with a weapon were 19.0% and 6.8%, respectively. Of these, 32.6% of the women and 1.9% of the men developed PTSD.

Whether or not post-traumatic stress disorder (PTSD) develops after a traumatic experience depends on many factors, one of which is the type of trauma.
- After a rape, 50 to 80% of those affected develop PTSD.
- After a non-sexual violent crime, approximately 25% develop PTSD.
- Victims of war, displacement and torture show PTSD in approximately 50 to 70% of cases.
- 15% to 39% of victims of traffic accidents develop symptoms of PTSD.
- People who suffer from serious physical illnesses (e.g. cancer, heart attack) also show PTSD in approximately 10% of cases.
- (Siol et al., 2001; Yule, 2001; Perkonigg et al., 2000)

Witnessing or experiencing a traumatic event can also lead to the development of PTSD.

In a study by Breslau et al. from 1998 (a total of 2181 subjects), 40.1% (men) and 18.6% (women) said they had witnessed an accident or act of violence. Of these, 9.1% (men)/2.8% (women) met the criteria for PTSD. 61.8% of women and 63.1% of men said they had experienced a traumatic event, 1.4% of men and 3.2% of women of which suffered from the symptoms of PTSD. Furthermore, the subjects were asked whether there was a sudden and unexpected death of a important person in their life (63.1% of men and 61.8% of women). 12.6% (men) and 16.2% (women) of those affected met the criteria for PTSD.

If one looks at how many people suffer from PTSD in Germany, it can be seen that this is approximately 1.5 to 2% of the general population. The number of those who have PTBS-like symptoms (ie those who have a subsyndromal illness), but not the full picture of PTSD, is likely to be much higher. Both a subsyndromal illness and PTSD have a very high tendency to chronify, that is, the symptoms remain unchanged or worsen if left untreated.

In a US study from 1995, people with PTSD were observed for more than 10 years in their course of illness. No therapeutic interventions were carried out in the entire observed group. Only one third of the observed people showed a significant improvement in symptoms after 12 months. The other two thirds still had symptoms of PTSD after 1 and 5 years. One third of those affected still had significant symptoms after 10 years, which restricted them in their everyday lives (Kessler et al., 1995).

2.6 The History of PTSD as a Diagnosis

The history of post-traumatic stress disorder as a diagnosis is, in comparison with some other diagnoses such as depression, a relatively young history, even though it has probably existed since there have been people who can come into traumatic situations.

Josef Breuer and Sigmund Freud described in their publication "Studies on Hysteria", 1895 a subclassification of hysterical disorder, which represents the late consequences of a traumatization. The German psychiatrist Emil Kraepelin, who created the foundations for the today's classification of mental disorders, described the symptoms, which occurred after severe accidents, especially railway accidents, as fright neurosis. The first investigations of a PTSD from a scientific perspective were carried out on survivors of severe railway accidents (so-called "railway spine syndrome").

During and after the First World War, returned soldiers showed symptoms of PTSD. The v people were referred to as "war tremblers" . After the Second World War, the soldiers who returned home also showed PTSD-typical symptoms.

William G. Niederland, a Dutch psychiatrist, described the mental consequences of the concentration camp inmates and victims of the National Socialist regime as survivors' syndrome (Niederland, 1980).

Many veterans of the Vietnam War showed the same symptoms as the soldiers after the First and Second World War. This was the occasion for a more detailed investigation of PTSD. Judith Lewis Herman, an American psychologist, eventually created the term of (complex) PTSD, after she had worked long with veterans of the Vietnam War. 1992 she published her book "Trauma and Recovery" in the United States, in which she writes about therapeutic work with traumatized war veterans.

In a diagnostic manual—that is, in the US-American DSM-III—PTSD was first included in 1980. This also marks the time when PTSD began to receive more attention. Research work and publications have increased significantly in the last 25 years.

PTSD was not included in the WHO's classification system, the ICD, until 1991, with the publication of the 10th version.

Friedmann et al. published the "Handbook of PTSD: Science and Practice" in 2007, the first compendium dedicated exclusively to PTSD.

The term trauma was originally used for physical injuries. Only from 1880 was this term also increasingly used for mental injuries.

References

American Psychiatric Association. (2013). *Diagnostic and statistical manual of mental disorders – DSM-5*. American Psychiatric Publishing.

Dilling, H., Mombour, W., Schmidt, M. H., & Schulte-Markwort, E. (Eds.). (2011). *Internationale Klassifikation psychischer Störungen. ICD-10 Kapitel V (F). Klinisch-diagnostischeLeitlinien* (5th ed.). Huber.

Friedmann, M. J., Keane, T. M., & Resick, P. A. (2007). *Handbook of PTSD: Science and practice*. Guilford.

Judith Lewis Herman, J. L (1992). *Trauma and recovery. The aftermath of violence from domestic abuse to political terror*. Crossroad.

Kessler, R. C., Sonnega, A., Bromet, E., Hughes, M., & Nelson, C. B. (1995). Posttraumatic stress disorder in the National Comorbidity Survey. *Archives of General Psychiatry, 52*(12), 1048–1060.

Luxenberg, T., Spinazzola, J., & van der Kolk, B. A. (2001). Complex trauma and disorders of extreme stress (DESNOS) diagnosis, part one: Assessment. *Directions in Psychiatry, 21*, 373–415.

Maercker, A. (1998). Kohärenzsinn und persönliche Reifung als salutogenetische Variablen. In J. Margraf, S. Neumer, & J. Siegrist (Eds.), *Gesundheits- oder Krankheitstheorie? Saluto versus pathogenetische Ansätze im Gesundheitswesen* (pp. 187–199). Springer.

Niederland, W. G. (1980). *Folgen der Verfolgung: Das Überlebenden-Syndrom, Seelenmord*. Suhrkamp.

Pelcovitz, D., Van der Kolk, B. A., Roth, S., Mandel, F., Kaplan, S., & Resick, P. (1997). Development of a criteria set and a structured interview for disorders of extreme stress (SIDES). *Journal of Traumatic Stress, 10*(1), 3–16.

Perkonigg, A., Kessler, R. C., Storz, S., & Wittchen, H. U. (2000). Traumatic events and post-traumatic stress disorder in the community: Prevalence, risk factors and comorbidity. *Acta Psychiatrica Scandinavica, 101*(1), 46-59.

Saß, H., et al. (1996). *Diagnostisches und statistisches Manual psychischer Störungen*. DSM-IV.

Siol, T., Flatten, G., & Wöller, W. (2001). Epidemiologie und Komorbidität der Posttraumatischen Belastungsstörung. In G. Flatten, N. Galley, A. Hofmann, P. Liebermann, E. R. Petzold, T. Siol, & W. Wöller (Eds.), *Posttraumatische Belastungsstörung: Leitlinie und Quellentext* (pp. 41–58): Schattauer.

Yule, W. (2001). Posttraumatic stress disorder in the general population and in children. *Journal of Clinical Psychiatry, 62*(Suppl 17), 23-28l.

Physiology of a Traumatic Situation

Contents

3.1 Why Feelings?—Basics of Emotions – 14

3.2 Acute Traumatisation and the Traumatic Pincer – 16

3.3 The Unbearable can be Borne!—Dissociation in the Traumatic Situation – 19

3.4 Early Intervention and Debriefing—Does Quick Help Help Quickly? – 20

3.5 What Protects?—Resilience – 23

3.6 What is at Risk?—Risk Factors for PTSD – 25

References – 26

© The Author(s), under exclusive license to Springer Fachmedien Wiesbaden GmbH, part of Springer Nature 2022
M. J. Pausch and S. J. Matten, *Trauma and Trauma Consequence Disorder*,
https://doi.org/10.1007/978-3-658-38807-2_3

In a situation where a person has to reckon with death at worst, there is a physiological non-reaction in the human psyche and thus in the brain, but also in the whole body. This reaction affects the thoughts, feelings, body and behaviour of those affected. Through these physiological reactions, "collateral damage" occurs, in this case changes, above all an incorrect storage of what is experienced during the trauma. This incorrectly stored will then become the symptoms of PTSD later.

The physiological reactions in the body during the traumatisation are, like the symptoms of PTSD, normal reactions. What is abnormal or was, is the trauma.

3.1 Why Feelings?—Basics of Emotions

Feelings are an important, even essential part of our human life. A life and further development of humanity and of the individual is inconceivable without feelings. Feelings motivate us, drive us, help us to recognise dangers, bring love, pleasure and joy into our lives. To assume that lack of feeling makes us stronger and more successful as well as less vulnerable is unhelpful and also wrong. Rather, it is about knowing oneself and one's feelings and dealing with them. Fighting feelings wastes resources. And these energies can be used more sensibly. Regardless of what each individual evaluates for themselves, whether they prioritize career or personal happiness, only a balanced overall balance will lead to sustainable success.

Excessively insensitive and too radical rational behavior can harm one's own goals and oneself. The environment, private as well as business partners, family, colleagues, customers, the team or the public can rarely guess or feel from which inner context and drive individual action is fed. As a result, renouncing allegiance and trust is not uncommon. However, from an individual perspective, the exact opposite is usually sensible, helpful and—if only unconsciously—desired.

From a biological point of view, feelings start important, automated programs in humans that have proven to be efficient and successful for survival and reproduction over the course of human development—completely independent of gender, location and social or societal status.

In addition, feelings reflect whether a certain goal or need has been fulfilled or not, and then provide the appropriate actions.

Feelings can be very intense or rather weak in quality. They can start suddenly or develop slowly; they can only last for a short moment or for a very long time; they can be experienced as pleasant or unpleasant; they can be experienced as well controllable or flooding.

In emotion research different basic emotions are described. These include feelings that are found across cultures. Depending on the author, these include, essentially, surprise, sadness, anger, fear, disgust, guilt and joy.

Our different feelings are like musicians in a large orchestra. If every musician plays at the right place and with the right intensity, it sounds wonderful. If every musician plays whenever he wants and how strong he wants, it sounds terrible. And so it is with the feelings too. In addition, it can be a problem if the consequence of a feeling is not desired.

3.1 · Why Feelings?—Basics of Emotions

Sometimes in the literature on emotions, a distinction is made between emotion on the one hand, and feeling or mood on the other. Emotions are characterized as occurring suddenly, being changeable, and having strong intensity, while moods and feelings are less intense and longer lasting. Emotions almost always have a relatively simple cause that is easy to identify, which is not the case with moods and feelings.

Stressful events and the associated feelings, such as grief, fear, anger, despair, hopelessness, have always been part of human existence. Such events present a challenge to the person affected. It is about adapting and perhaps learning new strategies for coping. It is about changing and perhaps discovering and developing abilities, strengths, and aspects of oneself that one did not know about before. Stressful events can therefore be the driving force for change, further development, and creativity.

> Only under the hammer blows of destiny, in the white-hot intensity of suffering from it, does life take on form and shape. (Viktor E. Frankl, 2005)

Do diamonds only form under pressure? Perhaps. But our own actions are an individual decision and the resulting pressure of suffering remains, even with previous, possibly incorrect, decisions—or lack of decisions—still within our control. The strength of the pressure is therefore regulatable. It does not have to be waited out until it has become so high that action is the only option and options are minimized. The timing and type of action are and remain an individual decision. It is by no means a weakness to seek professional help. This is just as self-evident in business life as it is on many levels, both public and private. A traumatic event is rarely truly avoidable, influencable, or predictable. But how we deal with it lies within the control of each individual. An actor in the public eye just as an exposed person in a position of economic leadership, both learn to sell themselves effectively to the media and make decisions of great consequence on a daily basis in upper management. For the sake of efficiency, profit optimization, or economic rationality alone, both would without hesitation advise not to close our eyes, not to wait for foreseeable negative economic consequences, and not to remain inactive in, at least theoretically foreseeable, increasingly growing follow-up problems.

The understanding in terms of reasons, connections and consequences is promoted in the following chapters and it is shown how adequate behaviour, whether from a purely economically oriented, private or combined perspective, can be based on knowledge. As a manager acutely affected himself, it may not be possible for him to take an objective view of his own status and personal needs in this period. So orient yourself to what you would do without hesitation in the context of a business decision: take things actively in hand, put your team together, open your eyes, face the challenge, go through it and see which of the resulting circumstances you can use to your advantage. This purely rational, profit-oriented approach as a first step will also enable personal development later on. There is no "wrong" except for stagnation and closing your eyes. And even that can be the right decision for a certain period of time for an individual. Because nobody but the affected person can decide what is right and what is wrong, as far as such a classification makes sense at all.

3.2 Acute Traumatisation and the Traumatic Pincer

When it comes to such essential things as survival, we humans of the 21st century have to admit to ourselves that we still function like our ancestors in the Stone Age. The reaction patterns and behaviour deep in our genes and our biology, in extreme situations in which it is a question of life and death, determine how we feel (or do not feel), think (or do not think) and act (or do not act) in such situations.

- **Subjective Life Threat!**

A traumatic situation is characterized by the fact that those affected experience it as an existential, as physically or psychologically life-threatening, or at least as a threat to health. In such a situation, it is of the utmost importance for survival that decisions about behaviour are made in fractions of seconds. Weighing in our cortex (cortex) would take much too long.

If you have your hand on a hot stove, you should pull it away as quickly as possible and not wait to think about whether it makes sense to pull it away or not.

In order to be able to react quickly, people therefore fall back on simple, fast and evolutionarily old reaction patterns in high stress and great danger.

- **Fleeing or Fighting? Dissociation?**

The oldest and deepest-rooted (namely, located in the brainstem) innate reaction patterns are **fleeing** or **fighting**. These reaction patterns are referred to as **fight or flight**. The two reactions are mediated by the sympathetic nervous system, the part of the autonomic nervous system responsible for activity. So whenever you have to flee or fight, the sympathetic nervous system is activated.

If there is no possibility of fighting or fleeing in the traumatic situation, only one ultima ratio remains for the psyche, namely the emergency reaction of dissociation. Dissociation means a freezing and a fading out or distortion of perception.

- **Our Stone Age Ancestor and the Traumatic Clamp!**

Let's take a closer look at an example of our Stone Age ancestor and the traumatic clamp.

> ▶ **Example**
>
> On one of his forays through the prairie, our Stone Age ancestor encounters a saber-toothed tiger. The Stone Age man immediately realizes that this is a life-threatening situation for him (**subjectively life-threatening event**).
> His psyche and his physical response immediately respond with the goal of ensuring his survival.
> The body secretes stress hormones and the sympathetic nervous system becomes active. His heart beats faster and his blood pressure rises, which increases his performance throughout his body, but especially in his muscles. The blood flow to the muscles is increased so that he is either strong in the fight or fast in the flight. He starts to sweat so that the body is well cooled in the fight or on the run. The breathing becomes faster to take up a lot of oxygen in the blood and thus in the body and to exhale a lot of carbon dioxide. The gastrointestinal tract is less perfused (digestion and food intake are completely unimportant in acute danger), which can lead to nausea and vomiting. The

3.2 · Acute Traumatisation and the Traumatic Pincer

pupils become wide so that he can see well. The attention is focused on the danger and everything else is faded out. Whether there are beautiful flowers by the roadside is completely unimportant for survival.

Emotionally, he experiences fear, anger, fear, and perhaps other emotions.

The body and psyche activate everything that is there in terms of energy and make it available, because it is about nothing less than the physical or psychological survival.

In the next step, the **attachment system** is activated as the first solution, so (attachment) people are sought who can help or protect. The Stone Age man therefore looks around to see if another member of his tribe is with him to help him. However, the traumatic situation is characterized precisely by the fact that **no attachment person** is nearby (rather, in many traumatic situations, the attachment person is even the starting point of the threat). The Stone Age man will now try to find a way to **escape** in order to escape the threat to life. But what is characteristic of the traumatic situation is that **no escape is possible**. As a result, he experiences helplessness.

The only way that would now remain would be **fight**. But if the saber-toothed tiger is much too large and too strong, the opposite is too powerful and thus a **fight is also not possible**.

The Stone Age man now experiences deep powerlessness and absolute vulnerability. This leads to freezing, a "freeze". It is switched to the absolute emergency solution in the psyche, the **dissociation**. The Stone Age man freezes and there is a drift apart of perception and memory. He only perceives the situation with the saber-toothed tiger distorted or not at all. Ultimately, this dissociation leads to the "playing dead reflex". This is ultimately supposed to make the danger pass.

The "playing dead reflex" has established and maintained itself evolutionarily because most of the "enemies" of man in the course of his development were not scavengers and would therefore not have eaten a dead man.

First, dissociation is mediated by the sympathetic nervous system and there is a freezing in the overexcitement. But then the switch is made to the parasympathetic nervous system. This is the part of the autonomic nervous system that is responsible for rest and inactivity. This parasympathetic nervous system consists of two parts, a dorsal part and a ventral part. The dorsal parasympathetic nervous system is responsible for the "totstellreflex", the ventral for relaxation and recovery. ◄

We have now spoken of the traumatic clamp bildlich the "thread" (life-threatening situation experienced) and the two "handles" (the two reaction options fight or flight) illustrated. The characteristic of the traumatic clamp is that the handle, ie the two "solution options" fight or flight, do not work.

▪ Incorrect Storage!

All available energy is provided, but nothing helps. And this is exactly the situation that is a super-Gau for our brain. Under these conditions of the super-Gau, the functions of the brain, such as reaction, processing, storage, memory, are only disturbed. Under these conditions, the storing of the information perceived in the traumatic situation does not take place in a "normal" way. These faulty processes are characterized by the fact that there is no (spatial-temporal) ordering, no evaluation and no structuring, which actually happens through the cooperation of different brain regions (Broca language center, hippocampus, cortex). The impressions cannot be sorted, named, structured and evaluated. Rather, the individual impressions are stored as individual fragments (i.e. images, feelings, behavior, body sensations, sensory impressions, thoughts) in a frozen state. This means that what is experienced in this situation is frozen in the state in which it is experienced in this traumatic situation. There is no processing, emotional reaction and networking with the other biographical memory. The memory of the traumatic situation remains as an active, acute here-and-now memory. So the affected people do not remember that there was a traumatic situation there and then, in which they felt like this, thought this and had these pains there. Rather, when they are reminded of the situation, they feel the same feelings, thoughts and body sensations as actively as if they were experiencing the same situation again. So the affected people do not remember, but experience the situation again as if it were happening right now. One does not remember the threat to life, but experiences it again. One does not remember the fear, but experiences it again. One does not remember the pain, but experiences it again.

This incorrectly stored memory is also often referred to as a trauma network. Every thought, every feeling, every emotion and every bodily sensation can only exist because there are nerve cells (neurons) in our brain that are responsible and active for the respective sensation. In 1949, the Canadian psychologist Donald Hebb described an important principle: "neurons that fire together, wire together" (Hebb, 1949), which can be translated as "nerve cells that are active together form common connections". The nerve cells responsible for the traumatic memory are therefore very strongly coupled because they are very active together under the activity of emotional centres. Through this common intensive activity, these nerve cells also connect very strongly with each other and are usually active together when there is an activation.

> ▶ **Case Example by Claudia S.: Acute Traumatisation and Traumatic Clamp with Dissociation**
>
> Claudia S. (name changed), 34 years old, is an internationally known film actress. She is divorced, was married twice and is the mother of a 5-year-old daughter with shared custody, which is repeatedly called into question due to her professional situation and the associated demanding time management as well as a "changeable lifestyle" that is imputed to her in a lump sum. She had no physical or mental illnesses beforehand.
> On a Thursday in November she decides, after the end of shooting to prepare for the following day, to stay at the set of an action film at the original location, a dark alley of a foreign city that is still largely unknown to her, and dismisses the driver assigned to her for the evening. When she leaves her motor home late at night, she is the last one to go. Still mentally in her role, lightly dressed and with only the essentials in her handbag on the way to one of the production vehicles, a man suddenly steps in front of her and points a gun at her face. The man screams at her in a language she does not understand, obviously gesturing, demanding money, car keys, jewelry and anything else of value she has with her. In addition, he yells, looking more and more uncontrolled, more unknown words. She interprets these for herself roughly as: "Or I'll kill you!"
> Claudia's heart is racing. She feels as if her heart were about to jump out of her chest. She starts to sweat, she trembles all over her body. In addition, she feels nauseous. She

can no longer think clearly, but only stares at the gun. There is only one thought in her: "I'm going to die now!" She feels powerless, helpless, panicked, hopeless.

Claudia's body reacts to the existential threat. The sympathetic nervous system activates everything in her that somehow improves the possibility of survival.

She does not want to accept the victim role, looks around briefly, hopes that there is still someone who could help her, whom she could ask for help (search and activation of attachment figures). But she is completely alone with this man there.

What could she do? Run away? She couldn't be fast enough that he couldn't hit her with his weapon. If that's really true—too high a risk. Fight? The man is almost a head taller than her and physically superior to her without a weapon. In addition, he looks drunk and very determined. The slightest hint of fighting him would probably be enough for him to just shoot. This is not a movie, it's real! She got herself into an hopeless situation. Should she say who she is? No, then the situation might escalate even further. She can't even speak the language! And what will the public say when they find out? Certainly that would not be good for her, the question of her complicity would arise immediately. Why is she dressed so provocatively in the middle of a November night ... And her daughter ...

No, there is no running, no arguing and no fighting possible! She is in the traumatic vice. Finally, she freezes. It's as if she were watching the whole scene from the outside. She dissociates. Suddenly she doesn't feel anything, she has no tension anymore.

The perpetrator rips her handbag out of her hands and runs away. Claudia just stands there. For how long? She doesn't know that afterwards. She only knows that it started raining at some point and that she found herself much later, soaking wet and hypothermic, but otherwise unharmed, in this alley. Around her are two strangers, one of whom recognized her and took pictures of the situation with his smartphone, while the other, correctly assessing the situation, just alerted the police. ◄

3.3 The Unbearable can be Borne!—Dissociation in the Traumatic Situation

Dissociation is the visual race of perception and memory. Dissociation is nothing fundamentally sick. Everyone has more or less the ability to dissociate. It is a neurophysiologically given ability that our psyche can use to cope with stress. Here, the psyche simply splits certain feelings, thoughts, actions, body sensations and makes them inaccessible to consciousness. The sense that lies behind it is that by this splitting an overflow with stimuli is impossible and those affected can better react and above all survive in the traumatic situation.

Everyone knows the situation when you are driving on an empty, long highway and then drift off with your thoughts. Suddenly you could no longer say for sure what was going on at the roadside in the last few kilometers. Or you sit in a boring team meeting and the colleague who always likes to hear himself talk again holds a long monologue about something totally uninteresting. Then it is easy to go to all those places where you would rather be now with your thoughts. If you are then addressed unexpectedly or even asked something, you have no idea what happened in the last minutes.

That's what dissociating is too. This ability to dissociate is different for every person. In addition, the ability decreases with age. Children in preschool and elementary school have this ability most pronounced. If you observe children of that age while playing, you can see this well. A elementary school child who plays robbers and policemen with his friends is also a robber or a policeman at this moment. Dissociation is therefore something that all people come into the world with to a different extent.

However, dissociation also represents a general human coping mechanism and is used in the event of stress, conflicts, crises, or similar. If it is a question of stress that meets the trauma criterion, i.e. the person concerned perceives a subjective threat to life for himself or others, then dissociative processing is even basic and decisive for processing. It is important to mention that the dissociation makes it possible to cope with the stress in the first place, but that no processing has taken place as a result.

A person experiences a threat where they have to expect their death, and they can't do anything about it (no fight, no flight!). This leads to extreme emotions within them such as fear, pain, hopelessness, helplessness, and many more. This unbearable state can only be made bearable through dissociation because it is kept away from consciousness. What happens during traumatization is split off behind an amnestic barrier. In this way, life can somehow go on. But two "states" also develop: the state with the traumatic memory (also called the emotional personality part, EP) and the state for "normal" life (also called the apparently normal personality part, ANP). If traumatization lasts for a long time, during vulnerable developmental phases, and is very severe, maybe even coming from important reference persons, then more than two states can develop. This way, multiple EPs and multiple ANPs can develop. If multiple EPs and multiple ANPs have developed, this is called a dissociative identity structure. An older term for this is "multiple personality." The ability of a person (usually a child) who was exposed to severe violence to develop a dissociative identity structure is to be called a creative and complex achievement. To survive in hell, the person had to adapt, and in this hell, it was the most reasonable thing to do to dissociate, because otherwise survival would not have been possible.

What lies behind this dissociative barrier is the traumatic memory, which can become active again at any time when it is reactivated by triggers, so-called triggers. Through these triggers, the memory material is flushed over the barrier into consciousness. The affected person slips back into the emotional state in which they were during traumatization and experiences the memory again.

3.4 Early Intervention and Debriefing—Does Quick Help Help Quickly?

After a stressful event or a traumatic experience, many people initially experience psychomotor agitation or a significant inner unrest. They experience fear, anger, panic or paralysis—often quickly alternating from one feeling to the other. There may be paralysis and a sense of numbness. The affected people withdraw socially.

These reactions are to be seen as normal reactions to an **un**-normal event.

3.4 · Early Intervention and Debriefing—Does Quick Help Help Quickly?

The affected people experience the complaints, the restrictions in their lives and the resulting suffering as abnormal. They may experience themselves as unable, weak and therefore try to hide the complaints.

Diagnostically, such a reaction can be classified as an **acute stress reaction** up to 3 days after the stressful event according to ICD-10.

If the symptoms last longer than 3 days and started at the latest 3 months after the event, an **adjustment disorder** can be diagnosed according to ICD-10. This may not last longer than 4 weeks, or 2 years in the subgroup of longer depressive reactions.

In both cases, supportive therapeutic support can be very helpful.

In the further course it then comes to a **processing** of the stressful event or a (complex) **PTSD** develops. According to the prevailing doctrine, this can sometimes only begin after months or years (so-called late-onset-PTSD). Here it is important that the ICD-10 deviates from this prevailing doctrine with regard to the time criterion and requires the development of symptoms within the first 6 months after the stressful event for the diagnosis of PTSD.

When considering the course now presented, two questions arise:
1. How can one help people who are acutely traumatized?
2. Is an as early as possible therapeutic intervention useful and if so, what should it look like?

■ **How Can One Help People Who are Acutely Traumatized?**

Early interventions are generally referred to as assistance and interventions that take place in the first 3 months after the stressful event.

For the processing of a traumatic situation, it is important how those affected peritraumatize (ie around the direct traumatic situation). Here, social support is an important factor.

Basic Rules for the Care of Acutely Traumatized People
- Convey to the affected person protection and security.
- Inform the affected person about what has happened, as far as this person wants to know.
- Important principle: What the affected person (does not) feel, (does not) think, (does not) do, etc. is NORMAL, that experienced is the UN-NORMAL.
- Explain the symptoms of an acute stress reaction and PTSD and show coping mechanisms.
- Try to activate the social network of the affected person as much as possible. Involve family, friends, acquaintances. The mere "being there" of familiar attachment figures helps with processing.
- Offer the affected person professional help. Give him contact details so that he can later turn to this help.

The two scientists Lasogga and Gasch have long been concerned with emergency psychology and have established some basic rules for lay helpers and professional helpers based on their research.

> **Basic Rules for Lay Helpers at the Accident Site According to Lasogga and Gasch (2011)**
> - Say that you are there and that something is happening!
> - Shield the injured from spectators!
> - Look for gentle body contact!
> - Speak and listen!

> **Rules for Professional Helpers at the Accident Site According to Lasogga and Gasch (2011)**
> - On the way to the scene, remind yourself what you expect and in what order you want to carry out the individual actions.
> - First get an overview.
> - Tell the victim who you are and that something is happening to help him.
> - Look for careful body contact.
> - Give information about the type of injury and the measures taken.
> - Expertise in the field calms.
> - Strengthen the self-competence of the patient by involving him in simple tasks.
> - Keep the conversation with the person concerned alive. Listen "actively" when the person concerned speaks.
> - Tell the patient when you have to leave and provide "psychological replacement".
> - Consider the relatives.
> - Shield injured people from spectators.
> - The helper's stressful experiences should be processed through relaxation techniques, individual and group conversations.

Is an Early Therapeutic Intervention Useful? How Should it Look?

An early therapeutic intervention appears to be useful if it helps the affected person to better process what has been experienced and thus prevents the development of PTSD. For the processing of a traumatic situation, it is important how the affected persons assess the consequences of the traumatization and how competent they feel themselves in the coping with the experience and the consequences.

In an early therapeutic intervention, psychoeducation plays a central role. In therapy, it is conveyed what happens to the soul of the affected person during and after the load. In addition, the symptoms that plague the affected person are explained in detail. The goal should be that the affected persons are experts on their symptoms at the end and that they have understood why and how these arise and what they can do about it themselves.

In addition, practical and sometimes also social support should be offered. At this point, it may also be quite important to bring in a social-pedagogical consultation.

During this ongoing treatment, risk factors for the development of PTSD should be explored and a closer look should be taken at the development of symptoms at each subsequent therapeutic contact. The aim should be that the diagnosis and treatment indication of any PTSD can be made early and then, with the affected persons, an individual treatment plan can be developed.

Under certain circumstances, a temporary medical treatment may also be necessary and useful.

Another treatment option is the so-called debriefing. This is a therapeutic treatment in which a kind of confrontation treatment is carried out very early. The treatment usually takes place in 6 phases.
1. Therapeutic goal formulation and information about the course of therapy
2. The patient describes the course of the traumatic situation
3. The patient describes the thoughts and impressions in the traumatic situation
4. The patient describes the worst moment (feelings, reactions, etc.) in the traumatic situation
5. The patient is informed about the symptoms, the disease and the course as well as about coping strategies
6. End of treatment

When you look at the studies on the success of such a debriefing, you can see that in many studies **no** post-traumatic disorder, in clinically significant effect, could be prevented (Bisson et al., 1997; Cuijpers et al., 2005; Litz, 2008; Mitte et al., 2005; Rose et al., 2001; van Emmerik et al., 2002). In some studies there was even an increase in symptoms (Hobbs et al., 1996; Mayou et al., 2000; Sijbrandij et al., 2006).

Because of this, a mandatory debriefing is not recommended.

3.5 What Protects?—Resilience

Not everyone who experiences a traumatic situation develops PTSD. Of those who are victims of rape and thus exposed to terrible sexual violence, about 2/3 develop PTSD. But this also means that in 1/3 of cases no PTSD develops. The victims of a car accident develop PTSD in about 1/3 of cases and in 2/3 not. Why do some get PTSD and others don't?

It is very important that it is understood why those who develop PTSD develop it. It is important to understand why this disease arises and how.

But it is also very important and highly interesting to understand what contributes to the fact that some people affected by trauma do not experience PTSD. Do these people do something different? And if so, what? If one could say exactly what these affected people do to avoid PTSD, one could also advise others.

This thought, which seeks the reasons why health persists or re-establishes itself, is called salutogenesis and lies behind the concept of resilience.

> **Resilience**
>
> The word resilience itself is derived from the Latin word "resilire", which means "to rebound". Therefore, one could translate resilience with "resistance to psychological stress". The opposite of resilience is vulnerability.

Since the 1980s/1990s, there has been intensive research in the field of resilience. It could be shown that resilience is not a personality trait, but rather resilient people are characterized by the fact that they can adapt well to the changing situations of their external world. They can expand their existing life concepts.

What Contributes to High Resilience?

There are factors that lie within the person and factors that concern the outside. Properties and abilities of a person that contribute to his resilience are:
- Experiences regarding self-efficacy
- Self-confidence and a positive self-esteem
- Social competence (empathy and taking responsibility friendliness, balance)
- A belief, or principles and beliefs
- A good education
- Presence of coping strategies/coping mechanisms
- Optimistic, confident attitude

External factors that strengthen resilience are:
- stable relationships and a good social network (e.g. family, friends, colleagues)
- supportive parents and carers, teachers etc. who encourage a realistic self-assessment
- cohesion and stability within the family

What can a person who has a high resilience do especially well?
- He can take care of himself actively and recognize, perceive and fulfill his needs.
- He relaxes regularly.
- He recognizes his own and other people's limits and sticks to them.
- He can make a perspective change and look at himself, his life, problems, etc. from different angles.
- He values himself and others.
- He recognizes that life includes successes, luck, joy, but also failures, crises, grief and pain.
- He can give his life a meaning.

It is therefore quite possible to increase one's own resilience. What is necessary for this has been gathered by the American Psychological Association and published 2008 10 possible ways to resilience:
- Make connections! (Have good social relationships!)
- Avoid seeing crises as insurmountable problems! (Make it clear to yourself that crises are surmountable!)
- Accept that change is part of living! (Change is part of life!)
- Move toward your goals! (Turn to your goals!)
- Take decisive actions! (Make decisions!)
- Look for opportunities for self-discovery! (Look for opportunities to explore yourself!)
- Nurture a positive view of yourself! (Nurture a positive view of yourself!)
- Keep things in perspective! (Keep things in perspective!)
- Maintain a hopeful outlook! (Maintain hope!)
- Take care of youself! (Take care of yourself!)
- (American Psychological Association, 2008; German translation by the authors)

> **Example by Claudia S.: Continuation of the Example**
>
> Continuing with the already presented case study of Claudia S., the actress who was attacked, the question can now be asked whether Claudia might develop PTSD and what she could do actively to prevent it. Her personal background seems unstable and burdened with a multitude of problems at first glance. But she does not necessarily have to be permanently burdened. Perhaps her daughter gives her strength and stability, maybe she has a strong religious belief or, precisely because of her exposed position, a particularly strong social network. Maybe Claudia is a very self-reflective or extremely self-confident personality, which makes it easier for her to deal with what she has experienced. Perhaps she is not aware of such aspects at all. Focusing on such inner and outer strengths and the support from the outside to become aware of such aspects is an important step, especially in the time immediately after a traumatic experience. In general, creating and maintaining such factors, especially in non-traumatized people and especially in management and public, is an important and thus also preventive aspect. As long as not acutely traumatized, much is largely controllable and even in complicated social or societal contexts it is usually possible for everyone to actively create corresponding structures and to reflect on themselves. Whether a physical attack or an accident, blackmail or robbery, nobody can be prepared all the time, theoretical thought games make sense. But as our case study shows, Claudia S. would have experienced the same thing if she had not been a well-known actress. So it makes sense to set up possible backups and options in the sense of the points listed above. If this has not been done and the person is already traumatized, these can still be established—or to become actively aware of them and to be pointed out what is already available. In any case, an active approach to what has been experienced is always to be preferred to a passive closing of the eyes. And if this has already happened, it is rarely too late to become active again. ◄

3.6 What is at Risk?—Risk Factors for PTSD

Under the heading of resilience, it has already been stated which factors protect against PTSD after a traumatization. But there are also factors that are considered to be a risk. If a person has experienced a traumatic situation, it is important to clarify which risk factors exist. The more risks come together, the higher the probability that PTSD will develop in the time after the trauma.

This in turn means that people who have experienced traumatic events with many risk factors should be observed particularly closely in the time after the trauma, so that the diagnosis of PTSD can be made quickly.

Risk factors that contribute to the development of PTSD are as follows:

- **Type of Trauma**

A first risk for PTSD lies in the trauma itself. The more severe a trauma was and the longer it lasted, the higher the probability of developing PTSD later on. In addition, the risk of PTSD is higher, the more life-threatening the victim experiences the traumatization. Another point is the cause of the trauma: If the traumatization was caused by a person, the risk is higher (so-called "man-made-disaster").

- **Gender**

Women have twice the risk of developing PTSD after a traumatization than men.

- **Previous Traumas**

People who have experienced one or more traumas in their lives have a higher risk of developing PTSD after another trauma.

- **Psychiatric Illnesses in the History**

If there were other psychiatric illnesses in the history of the people affected by the trauma, such as depression, addiction, anxiety disorders, it is more likely that PTSD will develop after the trauma.

- **Little Social Support**

This is particularly the case with peritraumatic support. If there was little or no support in the short and medium term after the traumatic experience, the likelihood of developing PTSD increases.

- **Other Stressful Events**

If there are further stresses after the trauma, such as job loss, legal proceedings, permanent physical damage, this also leads to an increased likelihood of developing PTSD.

References

American Psychological Association. (2008). The road to resilience. ▶ www.apahelpcenter.org/dl/the_road_to_resilience.pdf. Accessed 28 Aug 2008.

Cuijpers, P., Van Straten, A., & Smit, F. (2005). Preventing the incidence of new cases of mental disorders: A meta-analytic review. *The Journal of Nervous and Mental Disease, 193*(2), 119–125.

Frankl, V. E. 2005. *Ärztliche Seelsorge*. Deuticke.

Hebb, D. O. (1949). *The organization of behavior*. Wiley.

Hobbs, M., Mayou, R., Harrison, B., et al. (1996). A randomised controlled trial of psychological debriefing for victims of road traffic accidents. *British Medical Journal, 313*, 1438–1439.

Lasogga, F., & Gasch, B. (Eds.). (2011). *Notfallpsychologie. Lehrbuch für die Praxis* (2nd revised ed.). Springer.

Litz, B. T. (2008). Early intervention for trauma: Where are we and where do we need to go? A commentary. *Journal of Traumatic Stress, 21*(6), 503–506.

Mayou, R., Ehlers, A., & Hobbs, M. (2000). Psychological debriefing for road traffic accident victims: Three year follow-up of a randomised controlled trial. *British Journal of Psychiatry, 176*, 589–593.

Mitte, K., Steil, R., & Nachtigall, C. (2005). Eine Meta-Analyse unter Einsatz des Random Effects-Modells zur Effektivität kurzfristiger psychologischer Interventionen nach akuter Traumatisierung. *Zeitschrift für Klinische Psychologie und Psychotherapie, 34*, 1–9.

Rose, S., Wessely, S., & Bisson (2001). Brief psychological interventions („debriefing") for trauma-related symptoms and prevention of post traumatic stress disorder (Cochrane Review). *The Cochrane Library*, (2).

Sijbrandij, M., Olff, M., Reitsma, J. B., Carlier, I. V. E., & Gersons, B. P. R. (2006). Emotional or educational debriefing after psychological trauma Randomised controlled trial. *The British Journal of Psychiatry, 189*(2) 150–155.

Van Emmerik, A., Kamphuis, J., Hulsbosch, A., & Emmelkamp, P. (2002). Single session debriefing after psychological trauma: A meta-analysis. *Lancet, 360*, 766–771.

Symptoms of PTSD

Contents

4.1 Core Symptoms of PTSD – 28
4.1.1 Intrusions – 29
4.1.2 Hyperarousal – 31
4.1.3 Avoidance Behavior – 32

4.2 Symptoms of Complex PTSD – 34

4.3 Dissociation and Dissociative Identity Structure as a Result of Severe, Complex and Chronic Traumatization – 36

4.4 If Something Else Happens!—Comorbidities – 39
4.4.1 Anxiety Disorders – 40
4.4.2 Depressions – 44
4.4.3 Dependency Disorders – 45
4.4.4 Other Mental Illnesses – 48
4.4.5 Somatic Comorbidities – 48

4.5 Self-Injury and Suicidal Thoughts – 50

References – 51

© The Author(s), under exclusive license to Springer Fachmedien Wiesbaden GmbH, part of Springer Nature 2022
M. J. Pausch and S. J. Matten, *Trauma and Trauma Consequence Disorder*,
https://doi.org/10.1007/978-3-658-38807-2_4

After experiencing one or more traumatic situations, many different symptoms and complaints can occur. Often, those affected experience these symptoms as subjectively very burdensome. Sometimes, at first, no connection with the original trauma is recognized. Those affected may then feel that they are losing their mind. They may develop an addiction, become depressed, or suddenly suffer from inexplicable anxiety states. If those affected seek help, and only very few do so, they usually consult a specialist for the respective symptom. Someone with an addiction will see a addiction medicine specialist; someone with a physical illness will see their GP. Now the problem, i.e. the symptom, is described to this specialist. The previous trauma is often not told, because the affected person does not see any connection. Usually, only the symptom is treated, not the actual disease, namely PTSD. The reason for this is that trauma is not explicitly asked about in the medical history. So years can go by before the connection is finally made and treatment can be initiated.

Another variant is that the affected persons, perhaps because the symptoms set in immediately after the trauma, relatively quickly establish a connection between symptoms and trauma. This is often associated with the fact that the affected persons do not seek help immediately, but first try to deal with it themselves, or hope that the symptoms will disappear on their own. The affected persons experience themselves as unable in two ways. On the one hand, they experience themselves as unable because they have any symptoms at all. A strong, successful leader must be able to withstand traumatic events. Any other reaction is seen as a weakness. On the other hand, they experience themselves as unable because they cannot deal with the symptoms. A common thought: If symptoms occur after a trauma, then at least the strong, successful leader must be able to deal with them, that is, make them disappear.

Most of the time, the affected persons do not talk to others, perhaps even to others who have experienced exactly the same situation or a similar one. Too high is often the fear of being recognized as weak or even sick.

The affected persons live with the memories, the pictures, the fears, the constant tension. They avoid any memory, consume alcohol, medication, drugs to "calm down", to be able to sleep, or even to be able to work.

They experience what happens to them after the trauma, that is, all the symptoms, as un-normal and the traumatic situation is classified as normal; as something you just have to deal with. And exactly the opposite is done:

> PTSD is a **normal reaction** to an **un-normal situation**.

What those affected experience in terms of complaints is a physiological, normal reaction. The symptoms arise from the "faulty" storage of what was experienced in the traumatic situation. It was this situation that was abnormal and caused the brain to not function properly.

4.1 Core Symptoms of PTSD

PTSD is characterized by three cardinal symptoms, namely
1. Intrusions,
2. Avoidance behavior and
3. Hyperarousal.

4.1 · Core Symptoms of PTSD

To better remember these three core symptoms, you can use a little mnemonic device. Surely you know the three monkeys who cover their eyes, ears, and mouth. They have their origin in a Japanese proverb. Here they symbolize how one should deal with bad things: namely, not hearing them, not seeing them, and not saying them.

If you now change the hands of the monkey who covers his ears and instead has the hands NEXT to his ears excitedly back and forth, you have the mnemonic device.

The first monkey, who is excitedly waving his hands next to his ears, stands for overexcitement (one is totally excited and therefore waves his hands wildly).

The second monkey, who covers his eyes, stands for avoidance (one refuses to look and thus avoids any confrontation with what happened in the traumatic situation).

The third and last monkey covers his mouth but sees everything. He stands for re-experiencing; one sees everything just as it was during the traumatic event, but cannot say anything about it or about it. So you can't intervene and are condemned to re-experience.

The symptoms of (complex) PTSD can occur immediately after the traumatic event or with a delay (sometimes only after several years after the traumatic event) (delayed PTSD).

4.1.1 Intrusions

Intrusions are recurring memories. There is a re-experiencing of what happened in waking and in sleep, i.e. as flashbacks during the day or through nightmares at night.

Luise Reddemann and Ulrich Sachsse formulated it as follows in 1997:

> Intrusions are not memories, but re-experiencing of the traumatic situation: You are "fully involved" again, have "states", not reminiscences
> (Reddemann & Sachsse, 1997)

This makes intrusions very aptly described. As described above in the traumatic clamp, what the affected person experiences in the traumatic situation (all sensory impressions, all thoughts, feelings, body sensations) is stored unprocessed and unintegrated in a "frozen" state in the brain. This "stored" memory is often referred to as a trauma network. This network can be activated by external or internal stimuli, so-called triggers. External triggers can be, for example, the smell of a person or a certain place. Internal triggers can be thoughts about the trauma, but also natural bodily processes. It is often the case that the physiological reaction (e.g. the heart beats faster and one starts to sweat) to a physical activity (such as climbing stairs) reminds the brain of the traumatic situation, or triggers the trauma network (because during the traumatic situation the heart also beat faster and one was sweating), and thus causes a flashback. In addition, it can also happen that the trauma network is activated without a stimulus and that flashbacks occur.

During a flashback or nightmare, memories can occur in all sensory modalities. There can be images or films that run uncontrollably in front of the eyes of the affected person. But there can also be auditory impressions, so that one hears certain noises or even voices and dialogues. Not infrequently, the intrusion also affects taste and smell. In such cases, the affected persons have very terrible taste sensations in their mouths or smell smells that were present in the traumatization. Finally, it can also lead to re-experiencing of the body. The affected persons then have the feeling of being touched again, they feel pain, burning or similar.

> ▶ **Case Example by Ferdinand M., Part 1: Intrusions**
>
> Ferdinand M. (name changed), 54, married, two adult sons in college, a PhD engineer, is the chairman of the board of a German conglomerate with a number of subsidiaries in various countries. There had been no physical or mental pre-existing conditions.
>
> One summer morning, while on a business trip in New York, on his way from the parking lot to the main entrance of the local office and in the company of two colleagues, he is unexpectedly attacked by an activist, called a "capitalist pig" and attacked with a knife. The two colleagues intervene immediately and are able to separate the attacker from Ferdinand. The security personnel of the office building arrive quickly and are able to subdue the attacker. Ferdinand is injured by the knife in the neck and collapses. The emergency doctor who is notified takes Ferdinand after a short time, after his colleagues have given him first aid. Ferdinand himself can still remember the attack well, but has no memory of the time after. The first thing he remembers is coming to in the hospital. He has sustained a life-threatening stab wound, but is already out of danger by the time he wakes up and then recovers quickly. There is no expectation of long-term physical damage, he has been lucky again.
>
> In view of an upcoming board meeting and various important business deals, Ferdinand decides not to accept his family's offer to come to New York as well, and also decides against returning home immediately, even though his colleagues advise him to do so. He doesn't want to be deterred from his course. Show strength—both inward and outward. In addition, both his sense of responsibility towards his company and the worry of being replaced and possibly losing control are significant reasons for his decision. After a few days in the hospital, Ferdinand immediately and very successfully resumes his professional activity. He manages to leave most of what he experienced behind him. With full energy he pursues his business goals, which leaves him no opportunity to think further about the incident. A circumstance that is actually quite all right with him. And there is a little bit of pride involved—what a tough guy he is. No way—"capitalist pig"—let one of them try to do that to him. Immediately after the incident, his company took over the incident completely and after only a few interviews the legal processing can be carried out completely without Ferdinand's personal involvement.
>
> After a few weeks, Ferdinand notices that he feels increasingly exhausted, although he is used to sleeping little. In the course of time he notices that nightmares are increasing. Only after further weeks does he recognize a possible connection with what he experienced. With increasing intensity, the dreams go, although in different historical manifestations, basically always about the topic of the robbery.
>
> Although Ferdinand increasingly recognizes a possible connection, he suppresses such thoughts and hopes for the simple disappearance of the nightmares. He interprets them as inner processing that is now simply necessary. No reason to worry.

Approximately three months after the incident, Ferdinand is suddenly and unexpectedly jostled by a journalist from the side as he leaves a press conference. The journalist had stumbled over a cable and come unsteady. Seeking support, the journalist grabs Ferdinand and only just barely doesn't pull him down with him. This strong, unexpected, and lateral physical touch triggers a memory event, a flashback, in Ferdinand: In the same moment of the basically harmless event, Ferdinand sees himself again on the way to the main entrance of the New York office, the attacker with the knife in his peripheral vision next to him. Ferdinand is extremely startled and for a moment believes himself to be in a life-threatening situation. Only a few moments later does he come to and realize where he is and what actually happened. This unusual reaction is also not lost on his surroundings, but there are no consequences because the focus is on the fallen journalist, who needs to be taken care of. Ferdinand is drenched in sweat and his pulse is "180." Unnoticed and shaky, he withdraws from the event and tries to calm down. Although obviously not possible, he is sure he heard the voice of the knife attacker: "Capitalist pig." ◄

4.1.2 Hyperarousal

Hyperarousal is used to describe an oversensitivity or overexcitement. Those affected are in a permanent "on guard" position and always on the lookout for potential (life) dangers. A lot of energy is used in the brain at all times to ultimately ensure survival. In the traumatic situation, the brain "learned" that there can always be a danger to life. The affected person has a permanently increased level of arousal.

Physiologically, this overexcitement is responsible for the human amygdala. This amygdala, also called the amygdala, is part of the limbic system, and is located in the temporal lobe (so an amygdala in the left and an amygdala in the right brain). The amygdala is the "fear center" and is therefore something like the alarm system of the human and active 24 h a day to look for possible threats. This causes the human to be under constant tension, constant unrest, constant fear. Hyperarousal manifests itself in addition to these chronic conditions in the form of sleep disorders, increased irritability or even aggressiveness, but also timidity. Because the brain has to use so many resources for this survival security, only a small part is left for cognitive-mnestic abilities, which can lead to disorders of concentration and memory. Often, those affected describe that they used to like and read a lot and now have problems with the book flap because they do not know at the end of the text, sometimes even at the end of the sentence, what was going on before. Not infrequently, the affected then think that they are now also suffering from dementia.

The amygdala are not only the body's own alarm system, but are also involved in many other important processes. In addition to the formation of fear, they play a role in the processing of external stimuli, vegetative reactions and the analysis of dangers. Without functioning amygdalas, a human loses any sense of fear and aggression, which in turn leads to the fact that there are no warning reactions. Newer research reports suggest that they are also important for pleasurable and emotional sensations and are involved in the sexual drive. Monkeys, whose amygdalas have been removed, lose all fear and aggression.

> **▶ Case Example by Ferdinand M., Part 2: Intrusion and Hyperarousal**
>
> Since the experience during the press conference, Ferdinand has been alarmed. He is aware of the context of the incident, but he cannot deal with it and suppresses it, sees it as further part of a healing process that is obviously taking place. But Ferdinand is getting less and less rest. Nightmares are piling up, he rarely sleeps well, wakes up at night. He has not felt rested for a long time. At the same time, however, he feels extremely driven, restless, always in motion and action. He makes the need a virtue and uses the available energy even more for his professional success. He hardly ever sees his family, they seem more and more demanding and stressful to him at the moment. He is aware that such a flashback can occur at any time, that the actual event could also repeat itself at any time. As efficient as he is as a manager, he tries to adapt to the given conditions and be prepared. In fact, he experienced two more flashbacks in the following weeks. However, with different triggers, which increasingly leads him to want to be highly alert and prepared at all times. Gradually he becomes aware that comments from his colleagues may not be entirely unfounded. In fact, he is much more aggressive and impatient than usual. "But that's no wonder," he thinks, given the stress and also the working hours with the successes he achieves.
>
> However, Ferdinand increasingly realizes himself that his behavior, as reflected from the outside, actually costs him dearly. Unexpected slamming of doors can put him in panic for a short time. He also notices an increasing loss of concentration, which he can still compensate for well with the help of his team. In the long run, however, he knows that he will not be able to keep this up if it develops further. These nightmares all the time, hardly any sleep, flashbacks and always on the lookout—something could happen and his life could be in danger. Although he has this realization, the pressure of suffering is still not great enough for Ferdinand to seriously deal with things and, above all, with himself. He still wants to believe that things will sort themselves out and that this is just his healing process. ◀

4.1.3 Avoidance Behavior

If internal and external triggers repeatedly trigger intrusions, if one suffers from constant tension, it is understandable that any stimuli and apparently additional dangers and burdens are avoided. First, trauma-associated stimuli are avoided. The place where "it" happened is avoided. Similar places are avoided. If the traumatic situation happened on the train, one no longer takes the train. If "it" happened while driving, one no longer drives. In addition, one does not talk about the trauma, one does not even want to think about it.

In the short term, this coping strategy can also be quite successful. The tension subsides at first, one becomes calmer, the flashbacks do not occur and perhaps one has no fear. In the medium and long term, however, it will not be so successful. avoidance behavior is learned. The brain learns that situations, people, activities, etc., which are associated with fear, can be "solved" by avoiding them. Through this learning, a generalization effect (so to speak a spreading of the avoidance behavior) occurs. This means that the brain applies this strategy to everything that is associated with fear. But unfortunately fear is a constant companion of human existence and the spreading of avoidance leads to the fact that the social radius of those

4.1 · Core Symptoms of PTSD

affected becomes smaller and smaller. First, perhaps the place where the trauma occurred is avoided. Then large crowds of people, such as a Christmas market, are avoided because the many people there make them afraid and there is a fear that a similar traumatic situation could occur there. Next, gatherings of few people are avoided and those affected may only go into town to do shopping when there is no rush hour. Then specific time windows are sought in which there are particularly few people on the move, e.g. shopping very early in the morning. And at some point you order online. In the end, hardly anyone leaves the apartment anymore. The end of avoidance behavior is social isolation. But even there is no absolute security. There is always still fear.

Another form of avoidance, an inner avoidance, is emotional numbness. Here, any emotional reactions are avoided internally in order not to be reminded of the feelings from the traumatic situation. Inside, an emptiness arises, a not-feeling, so that one does not have to feel what one felt in the trauma.

> ▶ **Example Case by Ferdinand M., Part 3: Intrusion, Hyperarousal and Avoidance Behavior**
>
> Again, a few weeks have passed and Ferdinand's life has become even more complicated. What was a shock at the mere slamming of doors has expanded to all sorts of events in daily life and, in particular, to situations and moments that are in possible connection with the traumatic experience, that resemble it or simply remind him of it. Ferdinand is aware that something has to change, that he has to change something. But what? Go to the doctor? What is he supposed to do? He's not sick. And he's not crazy. And how is he supposed to explain visits to a psychologist? That would weaken his position considerably. Maybe a private personal coaching … But no, he can do it himself. And almost inevitably he comes up with the idea of avoiding situations that make him afraid, trigger flashbacks or favor his nightmares. And he quickly realizes: Yes, it works!
>
> First, he gets rid of press conferences and shortly afterwards almost all events where many people could stand around him uncontrollably. Not optimal, he knows that, but a significant reduction in the number of his flashbacks and nightmares seems to be justified. However, he still cannot calm down again if he is once excited. Memory disorders remain pretty much unchanged.
>
> But his avoidance measures are not enough anymore, Ferdinand increasingly restricts himself. After only a few weeks, it becomes increasingly difficult for him to meet his own standards in his profession. In principle, there is hardly any private life anymore. Ferdinand runs his company from home office after a while almost exclusively. By phone, Skype, online and without personal contact with other people. And even the daily commute, which he does directly after waking up and until shortly before going back to bed, becomes an increasingly impossible task. His family is now completely ignored. Ferdinand's quality of life tends to zero. His professional tasks, such as private obligations, can hardly be fulfilled anymore. Of joy, happiness and satisfaction can basically no longer be spoken. Until one day he also feels unsafe at home in his own four walls. Ferdinand instinctively realizes that he almost automatically represses more and more of any feelings, becomes deaf and insensitive in order to be able to function at all. To be afraid of nothing anymore. He has lost control. If he ever had it.
>
> At this point he makes a spontaneous decision: he gets professional help—as in everyday business life, to justify this to himself for purely economic reasons. But at least, because

he is clear: It is not about the business. But this economically factual consideration as motivation helps him. Everything theoretical and efficient, unemotional. So it can go. Ferdinand tackles the matter. ◄

4.2 Symptoms of Complex PTSD

People affected by severe traumatization, by traumatization that has lasted a long time, perhaps in young or even very young years, in sensitive life phases and caused by people who were important reference persons, usually show symptoms that go beyond the three core symptoms of PTSD.

Such people who suffer from complex PTSD also show intrusions, hyperarousal and avoidance behavior. But they also show other symptoms.

There is a change in emotional regulation with depressive symptoms, with anger, despair, etc. The feelings often occur uncontrolled and unpredictable and are excessively pronounced. The mood changes very quickly and there is a loss of confidence.

The affected persons experience a change in self-image and the image they have of the world and other people. Often they experience themselves as worthless and not lovable and they are tormented by strong feelings of shame and guilt.

Social relationships change very strongly. To some extent, the affected persons can build new relationships very difficultly because there is a very great mistrust. Often this change leads to social isolation, to mistrust.

In his book "Posttraumatic Stress Disorders" (2013), Andreas Maercker proposed the following diagnostic criteria for complex PTSD:

- **Trauma criterion:** The existence of a long-term traumatic stressor (e.g., victims of organized violence, domestic violence, severe sexual or physical violence in childhood)
- **Core symptoms of PTSD** (re-experiencing, avoidance behavior, numbing, hyperarousal)
- Impairment of additional areas such as
    - Regulation of emotions: Emotions are experienced as unbearable, uncontrollable, and there are frequent outbursts of emotion, periods of "numbness", depressive episodes, and self-injurious and suicidal thoughts.
    - Changes in self-image: The affected person experiences himself as worthless, inferior, bad, guilty and inferior. In addition, there is a feeling of shame.
    - Disruption of relationship formation: Relationships can be difficult to establish due to fear, mistrust, etc., it can be difficult to regulate proximity-distance, and relationships are often abruptly terminated.
    - Occurrence of dissociations.

> ▶ **Example Case by Norbert K.: Complex PTSD**
>
> Norbert K. (name changed), 39 years old, is a medium-sized entrepreneur and managing director of the family-owned asset management, which he took over from his father a few years ago. He is unmarried, no children.
>
> He has been suffering from sleep disorders and recurring phases of severe nightmares for many years. He can't really remember the exact beginning anymore. And he doesn't really

4.2 · Symptoms of Complex PTSD

want to. He has long since gotten used to the possibility of flashbacks. The fear that these events used to cause him can no longer be felt today. Overall, he is now an extremely unemotional, almost emotionless person. He has learned to avoid many possible triggers of his flashbacks. This is quite complicated, because he is not really sure what the triggers are and what they actually trigger—because he can hardly remember the contents of his flashbacks. Somehow it's always about sex. But, like a dream, it's forgotten shortly afterwards. He has largely made do with the restrictions that his avoidance behavior entails, considering his current situation to be quite normal. A strictly regulated workday with as many identical procedures as possible helps him. His apartment is on the same property as the office of the asset management. An assistant takes over many tasks for him. He doesn't really have a circle of friends, but he doesn't miss it either. His contact with his parents is also rather distant. Too many different business views, especially in terms of the management of the family business and asset management, are additionally in the way. He orders most of his shopping online and has it delivered. His former excursions into nightlife, with all kinds of sexual experiences, have also been reduced, he is not 20 anymore. Norbert is more feared than liked by his employees. Respect determines the interaction. Norbert's uncontrolled and impulsive manner, as well as his often extremely irrational seeming overexcitement, even if only small things happen, make cooperation difficult. With the exception of a lawyer who has been employed for many years and was still hired by his father, the average period of employment in the eight-member team of asset managers is less than three years: either fired spontaneously or voluntarily sought pastures. Norbert quickly delegated the direct and active work in the various companies of the family to others, which is why he hardly ever has to travel anymore.

In principle, in his opinion, therefore everything is quite normal. But he notices that he generally does not feel well, quite the contrary, he is often simply to cry and miserable. Not in the business, he has everything under control. However, he knows what everyone thinks: He is just the son of the actual boss. Worthless. Nothing of his own he has achieved. A necessary evil. He was born with a silver spoon in his mouth. But as soon as he leaves the office, he often can not decide whether to laugh or cry. Things suddenly appear as absurdly funny or sad, but in the end actually no feeling really remains. In principle only black. Nothing.

This black is sometimes so overwhelming that he can see nothing else. He does his job anyway … And often he wonders why he does that at all. He is not thanked for it anyway. He is anyway just the accomplice of his father. He always took what he wanted. What does he care about. Norbert? He does not exist. Only black. Black available to others. Yes, of course, his uncontrolled aggressions are somehow not good. But so far nothing has happened. At least nothing bad, nothing that could not be solved with money.

Occasionally, Norbert also feels an extremely strong sense of grief. Out of the blue. And not controllable. Unbearable. Too big. Often it helps him in such moments to hurt himself. Just a little with the knife. Just to feel something real. Something else. Something controllable. But also his work helps him to stay stable. At least a little. He can do that, he feels safe there. And actually he does that quite well. Even if no one sees it, the father does not see it.

Norbert has often played with the idea of ending his life. And often he has let it come to that. But no one noticed. Always everything went well. Also businesswise. Maybe that's one of the reasons for his success. But of course, also the reason for many setbacks. But even if that were the case, it doesn't matter. He doesn't get anything out of it anyway— he thinks—and starts laughing, excessively strong. Long and loud. After a while, his laughter turns into crying. He sits on the floor, crouches in a corner. Whimpers like a small injured child.

In such recurring moments, Norbert often can hardly remember the time afterwards. Hours later, he usually finds himself in another place in his apartment.

Norbert does not talk about all this. He lives with it, thinks he has it under control. He is ashamed, feels insecure and inferior. And who should he confide in? And why at all? ◀

4.3 Dissociation and Dissociative Identity Structure as a Result of Severe, Complex and Chronic Traumatization

As described above, severe, long-term traumatization can lead to complex post-traumatic stress disorder. Often such traumatization takes place in early childhood or begins at this time. These early years of a person are very vulnerable, that is, sensitive years in which a traumatic experience hits a still immature soul and a still immature brain. As a result, the consequences are usually more far-reaching. Unfortunately, it is also very often the case that in these cases the perpetrators are important reference persons for the victims. This leads the victims into the almost insoluble situation that this person is a once-beloved reference person and then gives love, attention and security, and at other times the perpetrator, who causes pain, suffering and humiliation.

It is essential for a child to receive some kind of loving caretaker. But if this caretaker is also the source of pain, suffering and agony, the child is only left with the possibility to split off this part, that is to say "to dissociate". As a result, the knowledge, the awareness and the memory of the part of the caretaker that causes pain remain inaccessible to consciousness.

These processes of dissociation lead, in the case of severe, long-term traumatisation, to the fact that the soul of the victim dissociates structurally, that is to say, in order to survive, different parts of the personality develop. These parts of the personality are parts of the soul, each with their own memories, properties and emotional states.

Every person has different facets or parts. These are referred to as ego-states. If you talk to your boss, you will feel, speak and react differently than if you were playing with a small child. The transitions and boundaries between these ego-states are very fluid and usually go unnoticed. In the case of people who are dissociatively structured, these ego-states and the boundaries between them are very pronounced. To some extent, the different parts are unaware of each other, so that people affected by dissociation often experience phases of amnesia.

The dissociative identity structure (DIS) is a phenomenon described over 100 years ago. And even today it is still a very controversial appearance. The idea that a human soul functions dissociatively and thus leads to a multiple personality structure seems to irritate many people, especially those who work in the field of mental illness, to such an extent that many doctors, therapists, psychologists continue to refuse to recognize that "there is such a thing"—despite the many scientific findings in recent years and decades. The result is that the affected people not only carry the memories of their severe traumatization and the symptoms of post-traumatic stress disorder with them. Even if they finally seek professional help, they meet people who tell them that the way they work now—dissociatively—is an illusion. They

4.3 · Dissociation and Dissociative Identity Structure ...

even tell them that what they did to survive the terrible suffering—to dissociate or to structure dissociatively—was wrong and is still wrong. And yet one would actually have to tell these affected people that dissociation was the best they could do because it was the only way to survive. To dissociate, to structure dissociatively, is a creative, strenuous and successful strategy not to die in hell.

The dissociative identity structure is characterized by the following characteristics:
- continuous pattern of dissociative functioning,
- deficient integration of consciousness in the areas of memory, perception and identity,
- the presence of at least 2 parts that alternately take control of behavior.

In DSM-5 there has been a quite considerable change in the diagnostic criteria. Up to DSM-IV it was necessary for the diagnosis of DIS that the switch (i.e. the change from one personality part to another) was observed by the diagnosing person. This is no longer required in DSM-5. It is now sufficient that the patient reports it.

Furthermore, up to DSM-IV, the described amnesias only applied to traumatic events. Since DSM-5, these amnestic phases have now been extended to phases of everyday events.

In the ICD-10 (research) criteria for the diagnosis of dissociative identity disorder (DIS; multiple personality) the following points are required for the diagnosis:
- 2 or more different personalities within an individual, of which at any given time only one is verifiable.
- Each personality has its own memory, its own preferences and behaviors and at a certain time, also repeatedly, takes full control over the behavior of the affected person.
- Unable to remember important personal information, which is too pronounced for simple forgetfulness.
- (ICD-10, Dilling et al., 2011)

Paul Dell based on the results of numerous studies on the clinical presentation of dissociative disorders develops a comprehensive diagnostic concept. This concept appears to be much more satisfactory than that of the ICD-10 or the DSM-5.

- **Diagnostic Criteria for Dissociative Disorders According to Dell (2002)**

Continuous pattern of dissociative functioning with the following symptoms:
- dissociative symptoms of memory and perception (at least 4 of 6)
  - memory problems, conspicuous gaps in memory
  - depersonalization
  - derealization
  - flashback experience (echo memories of traumatic experiences)
  - somatoform dissociation (somatoform or pseudoneurological symptoms, dissociative movement or sensory disorders)
  - trance states
- signs of the manifestation of partially dissociated self-states (at least 6 of 11)
  - hearing children's voices (localization in the head)
  - inner dialogues or disputes

- derogatory or threatening inner voices
- partially dissociated (experienced as not belonging to oneself at times) speech
- partially dissociated thoughts: imposed, intrusive thoughts, also thought withdrawal
- partially dissociated emotions: feelings are experienced as imposed or intruded
- partially dissociated behavior: actions are experienced as not under one's own control
- irritating experiences of changed identity: feeling or behaving like a completely different person
- Uncertainty about one's own identity (due to repeated self-stranger thoughts, attitudes, behaviors, emotions, skills, etc.)
- The presence of part-dissociated states: in the investigation situation, the part-dissociated state occurs directly, which indicates that it is not the person to be examined, but then no amnesia of the primary person

- For objective and subjective manifestations of completely dissociated states of self (at least 2)
  - Repeated amnesia for one's own behavior:
    - Gaps in time experience (lose time, "come to oneself", fugue episodes)
  - Non-reminiscible behavior:
    - Feedback from others about their own behavior that they cannot remember
    - Finding things in their own possession that they cannot remember acquiring
    - Finding notes or drawings of themselves that they cannot remember making
    - Hints for recently performed actions that they cannot remember
    - Discovering self-injuries or attempted suicides that they cannot remember
  - The presence of fully dissociated states of self: In the investigation situation, a fully dissociated state of self occurs directly, which indicates that it is not the primary person being investigated, followed by amnesia of the primary person

In several studies in North America and Europe, it was found that there are approximately 1% of people in the general population who have a DIS (Johnson et al., 2006; Sar et al., 2007; Ross, 1991). In a study by Saß from 1996 it is also shown that women were diagnosed with DIS about 9 times more often than men (Saß et al., 1996).

When looking at the group of people who were in general psychiatric treatment, it was found that about 5% of them had the diagnosis of DIS.

People with a dissociative identity structure often have a high level of functioning and are often very successful in their careers. Nevertheless, they suffer from a high degree of suffering, on the one hand through the symptoms of complex PTSD (flashbacks, hyperarousal, etc.), on the other hand through the complications of dissociative functioning. The treatment of people with a DIS should be in the hands of experienced trauma therapists who also have knowledge and experience in the treatment of people with a DIS.

> ▶ **Case Example by Manuela B.: Dissociative Identity Structure as a Result of Severe, Complex and Chronic Traumatization**

Manuela B. (name changed), 44 years old, is a TV moderator of various talk and entertainment shows, employed, with a good income. She is unmarried, has no children and has had no contact with her family for several years.

For many years, Manuela has been plagued by flashbacks. She can remember the original beginning well, but she can no longer assign it to a specific time. Over-excitement and avoidance behavior are part of her normal daily routine, which she considers relatively normal. She accepts the severe restrictions on her quality of life as given. The content of her flashbacks points to a possible sexual abuse in childhood, which she cannot remember, however.

In her professional life, Manuela is extremely successful and committed. She is highly respected in terms of content and expertise. The difficult personal dealings with her are well known, her sometimes almost irrational-seeming, impulsive nature is feared. But nevertheless she is very much appreciated by many people—both within her team and on the level of the broadcaster, as well as by the audience in her target group and the general press. Her personal weaknesses are forgiven her. But no member of the aforementioned groups has private contact with Manuela, professional and private life are strictly separated. Her fame and her good income give her special freedoms, so that this is hardly noticeable in general.

In private life, Manuela is rarely the moderator just described. This facet of her character is one of three personality parts that come together in her multiple personality. Although this would be possible, the three personality parts do not know or interact with each other, so they do not know anything about each other.

At home, Manuela usually lives the personality part, the facet of her character, the humble housewife and spends a lot of time compulsively cleaning.

If Manuela leaves the house for private reasons, her third personality part is usually shown: that of a ruthless seductress who picks up men from bars almost indiscriminately and with very clear offers.

All personality traits have Manuela's basic nature in common with flashbacks, overexcitement and avoidance behavior. Other expressions differ sharply from each other and cannot be combined in one personality. Manuela is not aware of this. She notes that she is occasionally referred to her very different appearance from the outside. But she understands how to explain herself, with the help of the personality trait "moderator" and its status. The missing lifetime, from the perspective of the respective personality trait, is difficult for her to explain to herself, as she cannot remember the experiences of the respective other personality trait, but this is no longer relevant. She got used to it. The risks associated with her personality trait "seducer", such as sexually transmitted diseases or violent attacks, she takes for granted, yes, to a certain extent she even wishes for and provokes them. ◀

4.4 If Something Else Happens!—Comorbidities

In the year 1995 Ronald C. Kessler et al. published the data of a large study on comorbidities in PTSD. Here it was shown that in 88% of the men and 79% of the women with PTSD in their life story a psychiatric comorbid disorder occurred

(Kessler et al., 1995). This means that in only about 17% of those affected by PTSD there is **no** further psychiatric diagnosis. So it is rather the rule that, especially in long-standing PTSD, there is another psychiatric disorder.

The most common comorbid psychiatric diagnoses are:
- Anxiety disorders
- Affective disorders
- Substance abuse

In addition, it appears that not only is there an increased risk for the development of additional mental disorders in people with PTSD, but there is also an increased risk for physical illnesses.

4.4.1 Anxiety Disorders

The probability of developing an anxiety disorder in addition to PTSD is increased by a factor of 2 to 4 compared to the general population (Gasch, 2000; Hüther, 2001; Pynoos et al., 1999). In a 1997 study, Breslau et al. found an anxiety disorder in 55% of 801 women with PTSD.

anxiety disorders are currently classified according to the ICD-10 classification system as follows:
- phobic disorders
  - agoraphobia with or without panic disorder
  - social phobia
  - specific phobias
- other anxiety disorders
  - panic disorders
  - generalized anxiety disorder
  - anxiety and depressive disorder, mixed

anxiety disorders are among the most common mental disorders. In order to get an overview of what is meant by the respective anxiety disorders, the following criteria are to be listed, which are necessary according to the ICD-10 to make the diagnosis.

- **Agoraphobia (Fear of Open Spaces)**
- Clear and persistent fear of or avoidance of crowds, public places, traveling alone or traveling with wide distances from home (at least 2 symptoms)
- Since the onset of the disorder, at least 2 of the below-listed fear symptoms (including at least one of the vegetative symptoms) must have been present together at least at one point in time:
  - **vegetative symptoms:** palpitations; heart pounding or increased heart rate; sweating; fine or coarse tremor; dry mouth;
  - **symptoms involving the thorax and abdomen:** shortness of breath; feeling of constriction; thoracic pain and sensations; vomiting or abdominal sensations;
  - **psychological symptoms:** feeling of dizziness, insecurity, weakness, or numbness; feeling that objects are unreal or that one is "not really here"; fear of losing control or of going crazy; fear of dying;

4.4 · If Something Else Happens!—Comorbidities

- **general symptoms:** hot flashes or waves of heat; feeling of numbness or tingling;
- There is a clear emotional burden from avoidance behavior or anxiety symptoms, and those affected have the insight that the fear is exaggerated or unreasonable.
- The symptoms are limited exclusively or primarily to the feared situations or thoughts about them.
- (ICD-10, Dilling et al., 2011)

- **Panic Disorder**
- Repeated panic attacks that are not related to a specific situation or specific object and often occur spontaneously. The panic attacks are not associated with special effort, dangerous or life-threatening situations.
- A panic attack has the following characteristics:
  - single episode with intense fear,
  - starts abruptly,
  - reaches a maximum within a few minutes and lasts for at least a few minutes.
- At least 4 symptoms from the following list (at least 1 vegetative symptom):
  - **vegetative symptoms:** heart palpitations or increased heart rate; sweating; tremor; dry mouth;
  - **symptoms involving the thorax and abdomen:** respiratory difficulties; feeling of constriction; thoracic pain and discomfort; vomiting or abdominal discomfort;
  - **psychological symptoms:** feeling of dizziness, insecurity, weakness, or confusion; feeling that objects are unreal or that one is "not really here"; fear of losing control, going crazy, or "flipping out"; fear of dying;
  - **general symptoms:** hot flashes or waves of heat, or cold sweats; numbness or tingling;
  - (ICD-10, Dilling et al., 2011)

- **Social Phobia**
- Either clear fear of being in the center of attention, or of embarrassing/humiliating oneself

or

- Avoiding being in the center of attention or situations in which there is fear of embarrassing or humiliating oneself
- These fears occur in social situations, when eating or speaking in public, when meeting acquaintances in public, when joining or participating in small groups, such as at parties, conferences, or in classrooms.
- At least 2 of the following anxiety symptoms in the feared situations at least once since the onset of the disorder:
  - **vegetative symptoms:** palpitations, heart flutter or increased heart rate; sweating; fine or coarse tremor; dry mouth;
  - **symptoms involving the thorax and abdomen:** dyspnea; feeling of constriction; thoracic pain and sensations; vomiting or abdominal sensations;

- **psychological symptoms:** feeling of giddiness, insecurity, weakness or numbness; feeling that objects are unreal or one is "not really here"; fear of losing control or going crazy; fear of dying;
  - **general symptoms:** hot flushes or cold sweats; feeling of numbness or tingling;
- in addition (at least one of the following symptoms): blushing or trembling; fear of vomiting; urge to urinate or defecate or fear thereof
- Significant emotional distress due to the fear symptoms or avoidance behavior; Recognition that the symptoms or avoidance behavior are excessive and unreasonable
- The symptoms are limited exclusively or primarily to the feared situations or to thoughts about them.
- (ICD-10, Dilling et al., 2011)

- **Specific Phobias**
- Either significant fear of a particular object or a particular situation

or
- significant avoidance of such objects and situations
- Common phobic objects and situations are animals, birds, insects, heights, thunder, flights, small enclosed spaces, sight of blood or injuries, injections, dentist and hospital visits
- At least 2 of the following fear symptoms in the feared situations at least once since onset of disorder:
  - **vegetative symptoms:** palpitations, heart pounding or increased heart rate; sweating; fine or coarse tremor; dry mouth;
  - **symptoms involving thorax and abdomen:** shortness of breath; feeling of constriction; thoracic pain and discomfort; vomiting or abdominal discomfort;
  - **psychological symptoms:** feeling of dizziness, insecurity, weakness or confusion; feeling that objects are unreal or one is "not really here"; fear of losing control or going crazy; fear of dying;
  - **general symptoms:** hot flushes/surges or cold shivers; numbness or tingling;
- The affected have a significant emotional burden through the symptoms or avoidance behavior and the realization that the fear is exaggerated and unreasonable.
- The symptoms are limited to the feared situation or thoughts about it.

The specific phobias can be divided as follows:
- Animal type (e.g. insects, dogs)
- Natural forces type (e.g. storm, water)
- Blood injection injury type
- situational type (e.g. elevator, tunnel, airplane)
- other types
- (ICD-10, Dilling et al., 2011)

- **Generalized Anxiety Disorder**
- At least 6 months with predominant tension, worry and concerns about everyday events and problems

4.4 · If Something Else Happens!—Comorbidities

- At least 4 symptoms from the following list (at least 1 vegetative symptom):
  - **vegetative symptoms:** palpitations or increased heart rate; sweating; tremor; dry mouth;
  - **symptoms involving the thorax and abdomen:** shortness of breath; feeling of constriction; thoracic pain and discomfort;
  - vomiting or abdominal missempfindungen
  - **psychological symptoms:** feeling of dizziness, insecurity, weakness or confusion; feeling that objects are unreal or oneself is "not really here"; fear of losing control, going crazy or "flipping out"; fear of dying;
  - **general symptoms:** hot flashes/flushes or cold sweats; numbness or tingling;
  - **tension symptoms:** muscle tension, acute and chronic pain; restlessness and inability to relax; feelings of being wound up, nervousness and mental tension; lump in the throat or swallowing difficulties;
  - **other non-specific symptoms:** exaggerated reactions to small surprises or being startled; difficulty concentrating, empty head due to worries or fear; persistent irritability; difficulty falling asleep due to concerns;
  - (ICD-10, Dilling et al., 2011)

In the treatment of PTSD and an anxiety disorder, as with all other comorbid disorders, it is important to include them in the treatment plan for diseases in order to ensure optimal treatment.

> ▶ **Example Case of Ferdinand M.: Intrusion, Hyperarousal and Avoidance Behavior with Comorbid Anxiety Disorder (Panic Disorder)**
>
> Ferdinand is trying to regain control by all means. He relies more than ever before on avoiding all conceivable triggers for his overexcited states, nightmares and flashbacks. But the whole thing is increasingly making him afraid. Whenever he believes to have everything under control, a new aspect, a new moment arises that triggers fear in him. Fear that increasingly often escalates into panic. It becomes increasingly faster and unclear what avoidable triggers are, because slowly but surely almost everything becomes a trigger. Or rather: No trigger is needed anymore, the fear becomes independent. Driven by panic attacks, Ferdinand focuses on controlling his fear as much as possible. The fear of getting afraid becomes almost stronger than the actual fear itself, which increasingly covers all other problems. A constant, sometimes more, sometimes less high feeling of basic fear sets in Ferdinand, which he can't shake off anymore. And pretty much everything around him, as well as what is happening to him, can be a trigger for his basic fear to spontaneously shoot up to panic level. Even heart palpitations, muscle cramps or other physical sensations become triggers for great fear because he experiences them as potentially life-threatening. Cold sweat, shortness of breath up to feeling of breathlessness, trembling arms and legs, blurred vision and other physical sensations are added. The information that Ferdinand has received after various and very difficult doctor's visits, namely that he is physically basically healthy, can only calm him down to a certain extent.
>
> It becomes impossible for Ferdinand to continue his work to the necessary extent and of the desired quality. He can hardly leave the house anymore. And even at home he can't feel safe anymore. Maybe still in one of his rooms, in his very own library. But not even there with complete certainty. He decides to withdraw, resigns his mandate and

withdraws into private life. This is where Ferdinand's family comes back into play. They recognize the situation and can now, that it is not completely excluded anymore, react and try to help: They organize professional help. ◄

4.4.2 Depressions

What is a depression? In the WHO's Diagnostic Manual, the ICD-10, 3 main criteria are listed:
- lowered mood
- loss of pleasure and interest
- reduced drive and increased fatigue

In addition, so-called additional symptoms are mentioned, such as
- reduced concentration and attention,
- reduced self-esteem and self-confidence,
- feelings of guilt and worthlessness,
- negative and pessimistic future prospects,
- suicidal thoughts, self-injury, suicide attempts,
- sleep disorders and
- reduced appetite.
- (ICD-10, Dilling et al., 2011)

In the last 2 weeks, 2 or more of the main criteria and/or additional symptoms must have been present in order for it to be considered a depression.

Depending on the number of main criteria and additional symptoms, the depression is then classified as mild (2 main criteria and 2 additional criteria), moderate (2 main criteria and 3 additional criteria), and severe (3 main criteria and 4 additional criteria).

The treatment of depression has 2 central treatment pillars. These are:
- medication treatment and
- psychotherapy

In the context of medication treatment, antidepressants are used above all. Contrary to a common prejudice, they do not make you dependent and also do not lead to a change in personality. Antidepressants lead to the fact that the metabolism in the brain, which is responsible for depression (e. g. change of neurotransmitters), is balanced again. Antidepressants have to be taken for about 2 weeks until they take effect. Sometimes, depending on the symptoms, other medications are used, e. g. sleeping pills.

In terms of its effectiveness, psychotherapy shows the same success as medication treatment, but it takes longer for the antidepressant effect of the therapy to set in. For this reason, a depression should always be treated both medically and psychotherapeutically.

Sometimes other treatment methods are also possible in individual cases, such as.
- light therapy (effect only proven in seasonal depression)
- wake therapy (you get up after half the sleep time and stay awake; as a result, the mood is better the next day)
- electroconvulsive therapy (in severe therapy-resistant depression).

4.4 · If Something Else Happens!—Comorbidities

For people who have both depression and PTSD, it is important to create an individual treatment plan that takes both disorders into account.

> ▶ **Example**
>
> Ferdinand M.: Intrusion, Hyperarousal and avoidance Behavior with Comorbidity Depression
>
> Ferdinand realizes that he has lost control, even though he fought against it with all his might and pulled out all the stops. He tries to continue as best he can. In his special focus on his work, which no longer gives him any fulfillment, he nevertheless manages to stay at least professionally successful. But he has lost any balance and any belief that the situation could change again. As soon as the professional distraction subsides, he only sees black. Although he still manages to continue his leadership position, albeit in an unusual and very limited way and almost exclusively in impersonal contact, he can no longer enjoy these successes. He increasingly only sees his failure and the end of his professional activity, his position, his reputation approaching. Then he would have nothing left. And that would be foreseeable. No matter how much he would try. Ferdinand slides emotionlessly and aimlessly through his life, unable to control it. He develops tunnel vision, sees nothing to the left or right, above or below. Only straight ahead, towards the downfall. Only black on the horizon. Quickly moving forward, his remaining strength fades.
>
> He decides to end his life on his own terms, resigns his mandate, quits his job. He is financially well off. At least he can go out with some dignity. He will explain it with "personal reasons, family, and so on". Whether anyone believes him is irrelevant to him. He thinks about suicide more and more often, surfs the Internet in search of ways to finally end it. With life. To accept the darkness. Ferdinand hardly has a meaningful sleep rhythm anymore, can hardly concentrate, feels worthless—if one can still speak of feeling at all. This does not remain hidden from his family. Although Ferdinand completely ignores this, they recognize his distress and organize professional help. ◀

4.4.3 Dependency Disorders

Alcohol dependence is the most common comorbid disorder in "traumatized" men (both war and civilian traumatized) (Jacobsen, 2001). The probability of developing alcohol dependence in men with PTSD is about 2 times higher than in men without PTSD (Helzer et al., 1987: 1.9; Kessler et al., 1995: 2.1). The probability of developing alcohol dependence in women with PTSD is 2½ to almost 3 times higher than in women without PTSD (Kessler et al., 1995: 2.5; Helzer et al., 1987: 2.8). Traumatic experiences in childhood and adolescence increase the risk of later dependence disorders by a factor of 3, in case of severe sexual trauma even by a factor of 5.7 (S. Kendler, 2000).

Why there is such a close connection between PTSD and dependency disorders is explained by 3 hypotheses.

- **Self-Medication Hypothesis**

After a traumatic experience, the symptoms of PTSD occur, such as re-experiencing, hyperarousal, anxiety, social anxiety and avoidance behavior. Perhaps certain social expectations in the profession can only be fulfilled with difficulty, if at all.

Meetings with business customers are experienced as insurmountable. Customer contact brings flashbacks with it. At some point, those affected realize that all this is somehow more bearable if you have had a glass of wine, taken a sedative or smoked a joint. In the meeting you are again relaxed and eloquent. Customer contact is bearable again.

With these substances, an attempt is made to bring the symptoms under control. This also succeeds at first, but then an addiction develops from this self-medication.

- **High-Risk Hypothesis**

Under this hypothesis, it is assumed that people who are already addicted have an increased likelihood of being traumatized. Due to the addiction, it may come to procurement criminality, in the course of which one has to move in a milieu in which violence, aggressiveness and boundary violations occur much more frequently. In addition, a person who is intoxicated is in an exceptional state. There is a loss of control, a loss of inhibitions and one is more likely to get into high-risk situations than in a non-intoxicated state.

- **Sensitivity Hypothesis**

Addictive substances have a direct influence on the human brain and affect the brain's processing processes. If there is now a trauma in the intoxicated state, this leads to the fact that the processing and coping with the trauma is also impaired. People who are exposed to trauma in an intoxicated state develop PTSD more often than in a non-intoxicated state.

So far, only the self-medication hypothesis has been shown to be statistically significant. There are indications that the other two also have some significance

So far, addiction or dependence has been mentioned more often. Therefore, it is now important to take a closer look at when one speaks of addiction or dependence.

The diagnostic criteria for a dependence disorder according to the ICD-10 are as follows:
- Strong desire or a kind of compulsion to consume the substance
- Reduced control over the start, end and amount of consumption
- Withdrawal syndrome (trembling, sweaty hands, heart racing, …) when discontinuing or reducing consumption
- Evidence of tolerance. The same effect is achieved by a constant increase in the dose of the substance
- Progressive neglect of other pleasures and interests in favor of substance abuse
- Persistent substance abuse despite evidence of clear harmful consequences (e.g. liver damage)
- **Time criterion:** at least 3 of the above criteria met together in the last 12 months.
- (ICD-10, Dilling et al., 2011)

The treatment of addiction stands on three central pillars:
- Detoxification
- Rehabilitation (Motivation)
- Relapse prevention (e.g. self-help group)

The first step in the treatment of addiction is a qualified inpatient psychiatric detoxification treatment. This lasts for alcohol about 14 days. From the first day, patients receive no alcohol anymore. However, medications are given which intercept the withdrawal and prevent dangerous complications, such as an withdrawal seizure. The duration of a benzodiazepine withdrawal treatment is significantly longer than 2 weeks, because benzodiazepines must be slowly, sometimes over weeks and months, weaned to prevent severe, sometimes life-threatening complications. The benzodiazepine withdrawal is therefore dependent on the amount of each consumption.

After the completion of the detoxification treatment the body is free of the addictive substance and there is no physical dependence anymore. However, the psychological dependence remains. The addictive behavior, the desire or urge for the addictive substance in certain situations, is still deeply ingrained in the brain. Whenever the affected persons come into situations in which they previously consumed the addictive substance, this desire for consumption will arise again in them. That is why it is important that in the rehabilitation treatment the way of dealing with it is worked on. In addition, strategies and behaviors must be established which come into alternative use.

Even if the detoxification treatment is completed, those affected are well equipped for a life without the addictive substance. Nevertheless, they will again and again get into difficult, stressful situations or crises. In addition, those affected are faced with the task of maintaining what has been learned in everyday life. The aim is to prevent relapses. The connection to a self-help group is helpful here, such as Alcoholics Anonymous.

For people who have both an addiction and PTSD, the following is shown in treatment studies (Brown, 1994, 2000; Ouimette, 2000; Abueg & Fairbank, 1991):
- People with an addiction and PTSD responded less favorably to addiction treatment.
- People with an addiction and PTSD have more frequent and severe relapses.
- The symptoms of PTSD interfered with the rehabilitation of addiction.

Therefore, in patients with addiction and PTSD, a combined treatment is necessary. This means, first of all, that all complaints and symptoms are openly reported to the treating physicians and therapists. Often, the trauma therapists are not told about the addiction behavior because it is very guilt- and shame-ridden. And the addiction therapists are not told about the symptoms of PTSD.

Only with a treatment plan that includes both disorders can the affected persons be helped in a meaningful and sustainable way.

> ▶ **Example Case of Ferdinand M.: Intrusion, Hyperarousal and Avoidance Behavior with Comorbidity Addiction**
>
> In search of relief and in the desire to regain control, Ferdinand realizes that consuming alcohol surprisingly helps him a lot. Not really a friend of alcoholic drinks, he experiments a little and uses the unhindered and almost unlimited access that his position and the environment he lives in offer him. So far, Ferdinand has mostly withdrawn when it came to drinking together and, if only out of politeness. Now he deliberately uses such opportunities and also lays in his own supply, which he can always fall back on should

unexpected situations or requirements—such as unavoidable press conferences—arise. Almost euphoric, Ferdinand discovers how good a little intoxication does him, how relaxing it is, how well it helps him to fall asleep or just to take a moment of rest. He has to avoid fewer situations or other possible triggers of anxiety, feels much freer, lighter, has a lower threshold of irritation, fewer flashbacks and, in general, feels much more balanced, simply better.

Hooked on this discovery, he expands his experiments to soft drugs like marijuana and finds that a little joint has a similarly positive effect. Controlling himself and well aware of the danger of addiction, Ferdinand deliberately and almost strategically reduces his consumption of alcohol. He distances himself significantly and consciously from other drugs. This is not for him, he doesn't need it, it's not appropriate for his position and experience. In addition, he sets the potential to possibly lose control as relatively high and doesn't even want to get into this problematic situation. He also sees a certain criminal component, which he can in no way agree to, as it could also make him blackmailable.

However, over time Ferdinand's threshold of excitement sinks and the amount of alcohol must be constantly increased in order to achieve the desired effect, which increasingly rarely, at least to the desired extent, works. Since Ferdinand's environment, mainly from the business sector, notices and supports the initially positive change, he gets caught up in a spiral, not being able to stop and gradually losing control. But Ferdinand doesn't notice that at first. The focus is on business success. After a while, Ferdinand realizes that he doesn't want it any other way. He doesn't want a meeting without consuming alcohol first. After a while, Ferdinand has to realize that it's not about what he wants or doesn't want anymore. He can't help it. But at this point Ferdinand doesn't want to think seriously anymore. He's glad if he can get everything together somehow. He's not taking drugs. Good thing he was so strict with himself. There is no longer any talk of his own claim and performance. It's increasingly just about functioning. His family has no chance to influence Ferdinand. He doesn't let himself be helped, he turns away. ◀

4.4.4 Other Mental Illnesses

In addition to the previously mentioned mental illnesses, those affected by PTSD also have somatization disorders, especially somatoform pain disorders, OCD and eating disorders, more often than non-affected people. It is important to also take these symptom areas into account in the treatment planning and to include them in the detailed planning of the individual treatment.

4.4.5 Somatic Comorbidities

In the context of PTSD, not only mental comorbidities, but also physical diseases can occur.

In a study over 22 years (from 1989 to 2011) a total of approximately 50,000 women were observed. 12% of the women who suffered from PTSD at the beginning of the study later developed Type II diabetes. Of the women who did not have PTSD, only 7% developed Type II diabetes. Obesity was probably responsible for the additional diabetes cases (2015). How PTSD is linked to weight gain is not yet

4.4 · If Something Else Happens!—Comorbidities

known, possibly high concentrations of stress hormones play a role. This problem probably also exists in men who suffer from PTSD, but this has not been sufficiently investigated.

> ▶ **Case Example by Ferdinand M.: Intrusion, Hyperarousal and Avoidance Behavior with Comorbidity Obesity**
>
> In his search for relief, Ferdinand realizes that eating has a very positive effect on him: short moments of calm and yes, perhaps even happiness. He is not really a fan of sugary foods. He also eats fats and carbohydrates consciously. With all his personal difficulties, he does not want to give up all the rules he has set for himself all at once. After all, he also has a certain responsibility to himself and the business.
>
> But driven by flashbacks, nightmares and sleep disorders, his eating habits now change almost automatically. Being aware of this development, Ferdinand still gives in to his needs. He thinks and justifies to himself: If he feels that he needs energy, that is, food, it can't be that wrong. At the same time, he realizes that if he doesn't eat on a larger scale and constantly, he can feel very bad very quickly and that in such moments even the smallest thing can throw him off balance. Not to mention the ability to calm down adequately again.
>
> So Ferdinand eats and gains many kilos in a relatively short time. At first he gets positive feedback from the outside world, both from his family and from his colleagues. How nice that he is doing better. They would be so happy for him. Ferdinand actually knows how deceptive this assessment is, but he increasingly suppresses such thoughts and tries to believe in the reflection of his outside world. At the same time, he covers himself with work to the extent that he hardly has any chance to think about something private at all. And the professional success, especially despite his enormous restrictions, seems to justify him. At first unhappy about the increasing optical change of his body due to the strong weight gain, he starts doing more sports. He quickly realizes that this can hardly be integrated into his everyday life. And it is also too strenuous for him. After all, he has enough stress during the day! So he resolves to eat more consciously and less, but he cannot succeed. The resolution only lasts as long as he has just eaten. But in the next moment it is impossible for him to keep it. He just needs the food. And he was never the thinnest anyway …
>
> Ferdinand finds a balance between food and fears, flashbacks and nightmares, overexcitement and sleep disorders, which he can cope with to some extent. His career is developing positively, but he is becoming increasingly overweight. After a few months, his family begins to pay more and more attention to him. He also notices cautious hints from his colleagues. But he has long since closed himself off from the outside world to such an extent that he can no longer deal with it. Yes, he even perceives this as criticism, as a very personal and deep attack. What do they know anyway. They should be happy that it all works out somehow …
>
> So some time passes until one day he notices new and unknown physical symptoms in himself. The symptoms of diabetes. Ferdinand seeks professional medical help. After an in-depth anamnesis, which gives Ferdinand the opportunity to open up at least a little, the doctor advises him to give in to his inner pressure and to seek professional psychological support in addition to medical treatment. He puts Ferdinand in touch with a psychotherapist, among other things, as part of various address suggestions. ◀

4.5 Self-Injury and Suicidal Thoughts

As part of PTSD, but especially in complex PTSD, there may be a so-called self-injurious behavior and thoughts of suicide. Self-injurious behavior means that either an emotional chaos and thus an unbearable pressure arise in the affected persons, or an emotional vacuum. In the first case, all feelings seem to occur together and the affected persons are no longer able to differentiate them more precisely. In this feeling chaos also shame, guilt, self-hatred and anger are included. This mixture of many feelings leads to an almost unbearable inner pressure, which can be alleviated to some extent by the person causing himself pain (e.g. cutting his arm, burning himself).

In the second case, the affected persons experience an emotional vacuum in themselves, they feel nothing at all. They do not perceive emotions, do not feel their body. This vacuum is then experienced by the affected persons as so unbearable that the way out is the pain that they cause themselves.

In the soul of complex traumatized often also parts are created, which are modeled on the respective perpetrator (so-called. perpetrator introjects). These parts think about the victim, that is, about themselves, as the perpetrator thought about the victim. The development of such parts, which runs through the so-called empathic learning, helps the victim to survive in the traumatization. The fact that the victim partly takes over the view of the perpetrator during the traumatization, which sometimes lasts for years, makes the perpetrator and the traumatization itself more predictable again, and this in turn gives security. As further literature on perpetrator introjects, the excellent books by Michaela Huber are mentioned at this point.

People who suffer from PTSD often have suicidal thoughts. If there is a comorbidity, these can be further increased. Suicidal thoughts are always to be taken seriously and should immediately motivate those affected to seek professional help. Suicidal thoughts can be treated and a medication can provide a quick relief.

In some cases, the "self-destruction" does not manifest itself in the form of self-harming behavior or suicidal thoughts, but in the form of a so-called high-risk behavior. Here, the affected people repeatedly seek out situations in which the probability of harming themselves is very high. This includes a promiscuous sex life, in which no attention is paid to adequate protection against infectious diseases, or the seeking of situations in which there can be an escalation of violence, e.g. in the form of a fight.

In the treatment of people with (complex) PTSD, the protection of life comes first. First, it must be ensured that the affected persons do not take their own lives or put themselves in a situation in which their lives are endangered. Because therapy is only possible with a living person.

> ▶ **Example Case from Ferdinand M.: Intrusion, Hyperarousal and Avoidance Behavior with Suicidal Thoughts**
>
> Ferdinand cannot decide to do something. He simply does not know what to do. To seek professional psychological or at least counseling support, whether publicly declared or purely private, seems unhelpful to him, much too dangerous if someone were to find out or use it against him. His position would be weakened, he would only be perceived as

unreliable. Ferdinand can hardly think clearly anymore, he gets stuck. There seems to be no way out, no alternatives. And it can't go on like this. Ferdinand's thoughts are circling and no longer allow an objective view. Advice from his family does not reach him anymore. He focuses exclusively on work, where he still feels somewhat safe. But this is also increasingly less fulfilling. In addition, he admitted that he is really not as good as he used to be, and criticism from his colleagues is increasingly taking its toll on him.

The thought of how hopeless his situation is, that Ferdinand begins to think about a conclusion, increasingly overwhelzes him. First more professionally, he quickly comes to the conclusion that, if so, it would have to be comprehensive. Suicide as an escape. What else? He is after all just a burden to everyone. And that would never change again. How could it. Ferdinand sees black. Confined in tunnel vision. No way out possible. In such moments it helps him to feel something. But it has to be strong. He begins to cut himself in inconspicuous places. The pain calms him down and another day goes by. For whatever. ◄

References

Abueg, F. R., & Fairbank, J. A. (1991). Behavioral treatment of the PTSD-substance abuser: A multi-dimensional stage model. In P. Saigh (Ed.), *Posttraumatic stress disorder: A behavioural approach to assessment and treatment* (pp. 111–146). Pergamon.

Breslau, N., Davis, G. C., Peterson, E. L., & Schultz, L. (1997). Psychiatric sequelae of posttraumatic stress disorder in women. *Arch Gen Psychiatry, 54*, 81–87.

Brown, P. J. (2000). Outcome in female patients with both substance use and post-traumatic stress disorders. *Alcoholism Treatment Quarterly, 18*, 127–135.

Brown, P. J., & Wolfe, J. (1994). Substance abuse and post-traumatic stress disorder comorbidity. *Drug Alcohol Depend, 35*, 51–59.

Dell, P. F. (2002). Dissociative phenomenology of dissociative identity disorder. *Journal Of Nervous And Mental Disease, 190*, 10–15.

Dilling, H., Mombour, W., Schmidt, M. H., & Schulte-Markwort, E. (Eds.). (2011). *Internationale Klassifikation psychischer Störungen. ICD-10 Kapitel V (F). Klinisch-diagnostischeLeitlinien* (5th ed.). Huber.

Gasch, U. C. (2000). *Traumaspezifische Diagnostik von Extremsituationen im Polizeidienst. Polizisten als Opfer von Belastungsstörungen*. dissertation.de.

Helzer, J. E., Robins, L. N., & McEvoy, L. (1987). Post-traumatic stress disorder in the general population: Findings of the epidemiologic catchment area survey. *New England Journal of Medicine, 317*, 1630–1634.

Hüther, G. (2001). Die neurobiologischen Auswirkungen von Angst und Stress und die Verarbeitung traumatischer Erinnerungen. In A. Streeck-Fischer, U. Sachsse, & I. Özkan (Eds.), *Körper, Seele, Trauma: Biologie, Klinik und Praxis* (pp. 94–114). Vandenhoeck & Ruprecht.

Jacobsen, L. K., Southwick, S. M., & Kosten, T. R. (2001). Substance abuse disorders in patients with posttraumatic stress diesorder: A review of literature. *American Journal of Psychiatry, 15*, 1184–1190.

Johnson, J. G., Cohen, P., Kasen, S., & Brook, J. S. (2006). Dissociative disorders among adults in the community, impaired functioning, and axis I and II comorbidity. *Journal Of Psychiatric Research, 40*, 131–140.

Kendler, K. S., Bulik, C. M., Silberg, J., Hettema, J. M., Myers, J., & Prescott, C. A. (2000). Childhod sexual abuse and adult psychiatric and substance abuse disorders in women. *Archieves of General Psychiatry, 57*, 953–959.

Kessler, R. C., Sonnega, A., Bromet, E., Hughes, M., & Nelson, C. B. (1995). Posttraumatic stress disorder in the National Comorbidity Survey. *Archives of General Psychiatry, 52*(12), 1048–1060.

Maercker, A. (2013) *Posttraumatische Belastungsstörungen*. Springer.

Ouimette, P. C., Moos, R. H., & Finney, J. W. (2000). Two-year mental health service use and course of remission in patients with substance use and post-traumatic stress disorder. *Journal Of Studies On Alcohol, 61,* 247–253.

Pynoos, R. S., Steinberg, A. M., & Piacentini, J. C. (1999). A developmental psychopathology model of childhood traumatic stress and intersection with anxiety disorders. *Biological Psychiatry, 46,* 1542–1554.

Reddemann, L., & Sachse, U. (1997). *Traumazentrierte Psychotherapie Teil I. PTT 3/97* (pp. 113–147). Schattauer.

Roberts, A. L., Agnew-Blais, J. C., Spiegelman, D., Kubzansky, L. D., Mason, S. M., Galea, H., Janet, F. B., Rich-Edwards, W., & Koenen, K. C. (2015). Posttraumatic stress disorder and incidence of type 2 diabetes mellitus in a sample of women. A 22-Year Longitudinal Study. *JAMA Psychiatry, 72*(3), 203–210.

Ross, C. A. (1991). Epidemiology of multiple personality disorder and dissociation. *Psychiatric Clinics of North America, 14,* 503–517.

Şar, V., Akyüz, G., & Dogan, O. (2007). Prevalence of dissociative disorders among women in the general population. *Psychiatry Research, 149,* 169–176.

Saß, H., et al. (1996). *Diagnostisches und statistisches Manual psychischer Störungen. DSM-IV.*

Dealing with Trauma and PTSD Privately and in Public

Contents

5.1 **Am I or the Others Going Crazy?—The Question of the What and Why** – 54

5.2 **Am I to Blame?—The Question of Why** – 55

5.3 **Break the Silence?** – 56

© The Author(s), under exclusive license to Springer Fachmedien Wiesbaden GmbH, part of Springer Nature 2022
M. J. Pausch and S. J. Matten, *Trauma and Trauma Consequence Disorder*,
https://doi.org/10.1007/978-3-658-38807-2_5

5.1 Am I or the Others Going Crazy?—The Question of the What and Why

If, after a traumatization, be it after days, months or years, symptoms occur, such as flashbacks, overexcitement or anxiety, then those affected first perceive them as signs of a malfunction in themselves. The affected people notice that there are complaints, that they experience certain "things" differently than others, that they can no longer deal with some situations that were no problem before in the same way.

The affected people experience themselves as sick. And very often they ask themselves whether they are now going crazy, losing their mind.

A connection with the traumatization may not be found and established immediately.

If this is then established, the thought may arise that others can cope with "something like that", only one can not, because one perhaps thinks that one is too weak.

People in public life, in leadership positions or generally active or passive in the media, are under high pressure and special requirements. A person affected by trauma or trauma-related disorder first of all perceives symptoms. But he may not associate them with traumatization. Under increased pressure, it is especially difficult to perceive oneself, to classify oneself correctly and to differentiate oneself from others. So perceived symptoms are often interpreted very quickly in relation to oneself or as a result of short-term external influences. A tendency to which a large number of people tend. The thought that one would go crazy is not unusual and usually very understandable. To create fixed orientation points at which one could measure one's own perceptions is particularly difficult under observation of a public. Sometimes hardly possible anymore. A social network, with sustainably trusted contacts, is in this case difficult to establish and maintain. So often only the trust in oneself and one's own assessment remains. In combination with the often enormous amount of information that has to be processed in such exposed positions and the many performance requirements that have to be met, this becomes increasingly difficult or simply disappears. There is simply not enough time and energy, as the relevance of the information is not recognized.

But if the connection between symptoms and traumatization is established after all, the thought often follows that "others also manage 'something like that'", "I am too weak if I cannot do it". The "something like that" is usually not really defined, because it can often not be defined at this point without further ado. Objectively speaking, terms such as "weak" or "strong" are wrongly set in this context, but for the person concerned it is often difficult to recognize this. Especially because the complexity of the process is unknown. People who can do many things at the same time, have a great overview, are widely networked and above all also carriers of responsible decision-making competence, it is often almost impossible to react correctly at this point. There is no fixed definition for "correct".

In any case, it is not about weakness or strength, but about inherent human needs and sensitivities that can be approached weakly or strongly, but say nothing about whether a person is strong or weak themselves. Although it would be a logical step at the point of recognizing connections to involve professional help, this is often not done. The worry that one might not be able to trust oneself is strong.

Maybe one is just weak at this point and needs to counter it with special strength. Or the worry about how the environment—whether private, business or public—might react. Putting oneself in the background is valued higher to avoid it. Someone might notice that professional psychological support is being used. Such an activity could be interpreted as a necessity, as a general weakness and used against me. It is not taken into account that a timely reaction controls the matter and, above all, solves it for one's own benefit. Ignoring and repressing, which is often the result of a "strong" approach, leads in the majority of cases to a lasting deterioration of the situation, which also becomes increasingly uncontrollable and leads to follow-up problems.

It is difficult to come to the realization that help is needed. In a comparable economic situation, professional support would be sought immediately—indeed, one would have to do so in a leading position in order to avoid violating duties and compliance standards. But this is not about a controllable job, but about oneself. The realization that one is the resource from which the successful activity in the job is fed and that this resource must be just as well cared for often falls short for many. The resource of one's own person is simply assumed to be given and infinite, often without seriously thinking about it. But it would be logical to become aware of this and, as a result, to take care of this underlying resource in a very special way in order to optimize all the resulting aspects. Such an inner reflection of oneself is one of the essential necessary skills of successful management. The dependent economic environment must be able to rely on the fact that you remain actionable and leading, for the benefit of all. As a result, it is not only a personal decision, but almost a duty to think about oneself and to act appropriately as soon as potentially serious problems arise. Just like in business life.

Whether this action now has to be communicated publicly is another question. It is not advisable to operate in secret and take the risk of being "discovered". But not everything has to be set out in public. There is always a middle way. As soon as the realization prevails that professional help could not do any harm, this should also be consulted. In your own interest. Whether this results in a long-term activity is not necessarily the case. But in most cases no damage is done. And even if, what would be the worst case? Nothing can be so bad as to get seriously ill and lose control sustainably. Go for it. No matter in which phase you might be.

5.2 Am I to Blame?—The Question of Why

After surviving the trauma, many people ask themselves whether they could have done something differently in the traumatic situation. Many considerations revolve around whether the trauma could have been prevented at all.

However, it is not only the question of whether "it" could have been prevented that often arises in the affected persons, but also the question of whether they did not deserve the trauma. Perhaps earlier traumatizations or neglect are reactivated and the conviction arises in the affected persons that they attract misfortune or are bad people and therefore deserve to be treated badly by people.

Questions such as: Shouldn't I have seen it coming? Weren't there any signs of the impending horror? Wouldn't there have been another way I could have overpowered the perpetrator? Couldn't I have prevented the accident if I had reacted better?

In the time after a traumatization there are many cognitive distortions and some cognitive biases, into which the victims understandably "stumble". We will deal with these cognitive biases in ▶ Abschn. 6.1.6 "Merry-go-round!—Dealing with thought circles" separately.

Asking oneself, especially as a manager or a public figure, whether one is to blame for experiencing a traumatic event as a trauma, makes very little sense. Nor does the question of whether one then did not "properly" deal with it and therefore caused oneself to develop post-traumatic disorders. Of course, one could have avoided the traumatic event under certain circumstances. Or one could have prepared or dealt with it better. Or, or, or. But what does that actually accomplish? First of all, nothing. No one is perfect and one cannot have this demand on oneself, even if one acts in many ways that are possibly quite perfect. One should not even try. In the context of trauma, it is about fears, about emotions. Of course, a lot can be trained and learned. But precisely strength consists in being able to react flexibly, spontaneously and humanely. This also on the basis of experience and training. But still human and thus always emotional to a certain extent. Expecting to be able to function exclusively rationally rarely leads to the desired success. The mixture is essential. And trying to completely channel and ultimately control one's own human qualities can only fail or come at the expense of mental health. It makes much more sense to recognize and learn to deal with oneself. Transforming resulting apparent weaknesses into strengths and using them as individual advantages that differentiate one from others, such as competitors in the market, is much more useful.

Asking oneself whether one has done something wrong, whether one is a bad manager, blocks and does not lead further. Asking oneself the question of why one is affected and not others, does not help either. Why not you?

Reflection on potential misconduct is always important, but can one actually distinguish between right and wrong in such an emotional field? Is there even a right or a wrong? Mostly not. Much more often it is often more beneficial to look ahead and consider what activities and means can be used on the basis of the gained knowledge to continue and be successful. So not to dwell on whether one could have prevented something, even if this might have been possible, but after the analysis of the status to consider how the future behavior can be optimized and the current situation resulting from the event can be approached constructively. Retrospective self-criticism is only useful to a certain extent in this context. To philosophize about whether one deserved to be treated badly is destructive and not very successful. Trust yourself. Not everything is suddenly bad. Act confidently, determined and future-oriented. This with adequate self-reflection and possibly with the involvement of professional support. This is strength and leads to sustainable problem solving.

5.3 Break the Silence?

There is no silence. Not even with a highly complex PTSD. Silence only protects the perpetrators, not the victims.

To talk about it usually proves to be a sign of strength. Whether it makes sense to talk about it is a question of weighing up the pros and cons. On the one hand,

5.3 · Break the Silence?

it plays a role in setting an example. On the other hand, it can stir up fears and lose trust, as well as strengthen potential enemies. Furthermore, talking about it also always means dealing with what has happened, and for that the necessary tools are needed so as not to be emotionally overwhelmed again. Showing weaknesses can demonstrate strength. In any case, it is important to create your own spaces in which communication restrictions are not necessary. And if this is only within the framework of an exchange with a therapist who is subject to the duty of confidentiality.

It must be regulated and adhered to where and when information is communicated. Misinformation is just as harmful and can be just as threatening or even backfire as not giving out any information at all.

All aspects behave in exactly the same way as in public or economic crisis management . The public in the press or on the Internet, for example in the field of social media, is quickly clever, increasingly educated and does not forget. Everyone can express themselves on everything immediately. With every criticism, every attack, however stupid it may be, one must expect reactions. And at the same time also with corresponding reactions, with an own dynamics, which has long since nothing to do with you anymore.

You don't have to react to everything and by no means accept reactions personally or even as possibly deserved. Nobody can know how the person affected, you, really feels. No one is entitled to judge, no one can evaluate. In the end, this can only ever be done by the person affected themselves.

But he can determine the content and pace of his communication to the outside. So if communication to the outside, then planned, addressed to defined relevant and previously determined target groups and consistently handled. Here you should not make any avoidable mistakes, perhaps even involve a specialist only for this area of public communication, without salami tactics, in order not to get into a defensive position at all and then have to explain.

Active communication is essential. Whether it contains the true and really relevant content for the person concerned is secondary, as long as this person has his own unrestricted communication channel. Public addressing of PTSD can be very helpful, but does not have to. It can be liberating and goal-oriented, but does not have to. The right measure, the right format or the right platform determine the success. But no alternative is to close your eyes; to sit out the things that may come, to be silent or even to give up and to retreat into your own personal retreat.

Trauma Coping and Professional Services

Contents

6.1 What Can I Do Myself—Strategies for "Self-Therapeutic" Help – 61
6.1.1 If the Memory Keeps Coming Back!—Dealing with Flashbacks, Nightmares, Traumatic Memories – 61
6.1.2 Not the Same Thing Again!—Dealing with Avoidance Behavior – 65
6.1.3 Always under Pressure!—Dealing with Hyperarousal – 67
6.1.4 When Half the Day is Missing!—Dealing with Dissociations – 72
6.1.5 When the Mind Falls into the Trap!—The 10 Most Important Cognitive PTSD Traps – 74
6.1.6 Thought Carousel!—Dealing with Thought Circles – 77
6.1.7 When Fears Determine Life!—Dealing with Fears – 78
6.1.8 What to Do about Pain? – 79
6.1.9 When the Night Becomes Day!—Dealing with Sleep Disorders – 80
6.1.10 When Addiction has You in its Grip!—Dealing with Addiction – 81

6.2 Resources – 81

6.3 General Basics of Trauma Therapy – 82

6.4 Behavioral, Psychodynamic and Trauma-Specific Approaches – 84
6.4.1 Stabilization Phase – 85
6.4.2 Confrontation Phase – 89
6.4.3 Reorientation Phase – 89

© The Author(s), under exclusive license to Springer Fachmedien Wiesbaden GmbH, part of Springer Nature 2022
M. J. Pausch and S. J. Matten, *Trauma and Trauma Consequence Disorder*,
https://doi.org/10.1007/978-3-658-38807-2_6

6.5 **Confrontation Procedures – 90**
6.5.1 EMDR – 90
6.5.2 Narrative Exposure Therapy (NET) – 91
6.5.3 PITT and Observer Technique – 91
6.5.4 IRRT – 93

6.6 **Medication – 93**

References – 94

First, those strategies should be carried out which can be carried out by the affected persons themselves. These are strategies that facilitate the dealing with the symptoms. Many of these strategies are also used in the context of psychotherapeutic treatment. Which psychotraumatic treatment options there are, will be explained in more detail.

6.1 What Can I Do Myself—Strategies for "Self-Therapeutic" Help

The mentioned "self-therapeutic" aids should support the better handling of the symptoms of PTSD. They are listed below according to symptoms.

6.1.1 If the Memory Keeps Coming Back!—Dealing with Flashbacks, Nightmares, Traumatic Memories

By intrusions people affected by PTSD are repeatedly, more or less involuntarily, in the situation that they relive the traumatic experience again and again, partly or as a whole, in images, films, emotions, thoughts, body experience. And not as a memory, but actually as a re-experience. The impressions and the feelings from the traumatic situation are experienced by the affected persons in the flashback as if they were taking place right now. These flashbacks can be activated by external (e.g. a smell or a noise) or internal (e.g. a thought about the trauma or a similar pain as in the trauma) triggers. Flashbacks can affect all sensory modalities, only one, several or all together.

Those affected experience falling into a flashback as something that happens from one second to the next. On closer inspection and exploration, however, it can be seen that there are quite typical symptom chains that lead to the flashback. This means that there are precursors, so-called prodromi. These precursors occur very often in a certain, almost always the same order. Often they are barely noticeable at first. In order to be able to better identify these prodromi, it is necessary to analyze each situation in which a flashback apparently occurred unexpectedly. This makes more and more of these prodromi recognizable. Because the precursors that could be worked out in the last analysis are much better and more intense in the next situation. In addition, the view for further precursors is widened. In this way, a very individual precursor chain can be worked out for certain flashbacks. The better the affected person knows them, the sooner he can take action against certain anti-flashback strategies.

When analyzing a situation that has taken place and identifying it, the following procedure should be followed:
- First, **sufficient stability and safety** should be achieved after the last flashback. As long as this is not the case, no situational / behavioral analysis should take place, but rather work should continue on stability.
- Then it should be clarified how the flashback was perceived, that is, which **sensory modalities** were affected. (See? Hear? Smell? Taste? Physical perceptions?)
- **Where** did the flashback take place? (Place? Environment? Other people present? What did they say, do …?)

- **When** did the flashbacks take place? (Time? Time of day? Was it dark?)
- What was the person just **doing** / saying? (Describe behavior in the situation exactly.)
- How did the person feel **about it**? (Stressed? Tense?)
- What is the last thing the person can remember before the flashback came?
- What was before? And before? (Here you can now begin to work out the chain.)

The analysis should be created in writing and be consulted again with each next analysis.

The affected are often very surprised that there are so many precursors that announce a flashback. There is also security when you know that it does not come out of the blue.

But it is also always important to note that you can carry out so many analyses, it can always happen again that a flashback comes unexpectedly.

If now the precursors and the individual flashback chain are well known, perhaps even noted on a index card so that you can always fall back on it if necessary, then it is important to have strategies to break this chain. The earlier you recognize the chain, the easier it is to break.

- **Counter Stimuli (Skills)**

On each level of sensory modality, counter stimuli can be set to the respective intrusive experience. These counter stimuli should convey to the brain that one perception (intrusion) belongs to the there and then and the other perception (counter stimulus) takes place here and now.

If the intrusion is a smell, it makes sense to have a counter smell in a small bottle. This smell can also be applied to a scarf or the collar of a jacket, so that smelling it is more inconspicuous. With particularly intense smells you can also rub Tiger Balm under your nose.

Taste intrusions can be interrupted well by intensive candy or sharp gummy bears (available in special stores for gummy bears).

The acoustic intrusions can be suppressed by either concentrating very precisely on the noises in the current environment, or concentrating precisely on what the conversation partner is saying. Another possibility, if this is allowed by the situation, is to put headphones in your ears and listen to music. The music you then listen to should be well chosen in advance. Not every type of music is good in this situation. The music should lead to the fact that the here and now can be better perceived.

An exercise that can be used for all intrusions is the 3-2-1 exercise. This exercise makes it possible to break away from the intrusive memory and turn to the here and now.

3-2-1 Exercise
Just look around you in your current environment. Take everything in consciously and clearly.
Now name in your mind
first 3 things you see,

6.1 · What Can I Do Myself—Strategies …

then 3 things you hear,
then 3 things you feel.
Breathe in and out consciously once.
Now look for 2 new things you see,
then 2 new things you hear,
then 2 new things you feel.
Breathe in and out consciously once again.
Finally, look for 1 new thing you see,
then 1 new thing you hear,
then 1 new thing you feel.
Breathe in and out consciously.
This exercise is not only suitable for distancing oneself from intrusive memories, but also for wonderfully ending thoughts that keep recurring. In addition, very good results can be achieved with the exercise when breaking through a panic attack. It also helps to anchor oneself better in the here and now if one is very dissociative.

As an alternative to the 3-2-1 exercise, a mental arithmetic exercise can also be used to avert the flashback. For this you can, for example, do the 100-minus-7 exercise.

100-Minus-7-Exercise
Take 100 and subtract 7. What do you get then?—Answer: 93.
Then calculate 93 minus 7. What do you get then?—Answer: 86.
Then calculate 86 minus 7. What do you get then?—Answer: 79.
Then calculate 79 minus 7. What do you get then?—Answer: 72.
Continue like this until you get to 2.
If you are still close to the flashback, start over from the beginning.
If mathematics is not one's strong suit, this exercise can also be done well with the alphabet. Simply say the alphabet backwards, starting with Z.

Alphabet-Exercise
Say the alphabet from Z to A. So Z – Y – X – W – V – U – … – C – B – A.

Reality Check
In addition to these distancing techniques, the principle of reality control is also helpful. This simply involves recognizing in a situation that may remind one of the traumatic situation, what is different in the here and now than there and then. If it is a person, pay attention to what is different about this person than the person then (hair? Glasses? Beard? Clothing?).

Screen Exercise

Flashbacks often come in the form of pictures or movies. With some therapeutic guidance and practice, it is quite possible to actively intervene in this visual re-experience. For this purpose, the idea that the images / movies run on a screen or television can help. This projected image can now be changed. It can be stopped, like with a remote control. The images can be made smaller, the color can be removed, the sound can be turned off, or the voices can be distorted. In order to create a distance, the idea can also help that one is only an observer and not a participant, as in a cinema or theater. In addition, you can always pull the curtain in front of the screen and thus achieve distance. These distancing techniques are very helpful if they are well practiced at first. But this often requires therapeutic help.

Safe Exercise

After a flashback or nightmare, or regardless, often memories and thoughts of the trauma occur, which keep recurring. To "get rid of" them, the imagination exercise of the safe has proven effective. Here you imagine a safe, or a large box, a cabinet—something that stands for a safe place of storage in the imagination. There you now pack the pictures, thoughts, memories that keep recurring. Then the safe, or whatever, is safely locked. Maybe the safe is equipped with a combination lock? Or with a lock with voice recognition, so that only the owner can open the safe with his voice. Maybe it is additionally secured with a chain or rope? Then this safe or this box can also be brought to a safe place to which only the owner has access. Here the imagination knows no bounds.

After the memory and thoughts have been safely stored there, it is usually the case that they reappear after two to three seconds.

This exercise takes practice. And that's why it's necessary to pack the memories and thoughts away again and again until it works. And it will work, it's just necessary to be patient.

The exercise is not about locking these thoughts away forever. It is about the affected people making the decision again when and where to deal with certain thoughts and memories.

Create a safe, a box, a cabinet or something else as a place where you can store thoughts, memories, pictures (in the form of photos), movies (in the form of cassettes, SD cards, or similar) or similar when they keep recurring.

Pack everything you don't want or can't deal with right now.

Tell yourself and the things you pack away that you are not packing them away forever, but only until the time is ripe, the space is created and you are strong and stable enough.

Secure your safe, or box, or whatever, e.g. with a lock, a chain, a rope.

Take further security measures that are important to you.

Place the safe etc. in a place that is safe for you and to which perhaps only you have access.

Repeat the exercise over and over again. It will eventually succeed and be a helpful strategy for you.

6.1 · What Can I Do Myself—Strategies ...

There are many more strategies for dealing with intrusive memories that come to mind. Only some are mentioned here. In the end, it is about each and every affected person developing an individual and effective repertoire of effective strategies.

But finding the strategies is only the first part, the second, equally important part is practicing. Without practice, not a single strategy can be successful.

In the end, there is still exposure therapy (more on this below). The intrusions arise from the incorrect storage of the impressions in the traumatic situation. Through exposure therapy, this storage is corrected and thus no intrusions occur.

The above exercises can be carried out in a short time and in many places. They are therefore particularly suitable for people in public life, in management and in the media. Whether in a hotel, an airplane, a motorhome on the set of a film or at home, fifteen minutes can also be set up between two telephone appointments in an emergency. There are therefore no implementation possibilities. The question arises as to whether such an exercise is feasible in terms of content. This is a question of repetition and concentration. At the beginning it is not easy, but after a few attempts it is successfully established in most cases, provided that the inner resistance to such an exercise is also overcome. In this respect, it is often helpful to realize that this exercise does not have to be done, but that it makes sense to want to do this exercise, that it does you good and creates individual freedom. It is not a task that has to be completed, like work requirements, for example. It does you good. Try to take it seriously. Give yourself such a freedom that you can sell it to others, for example, as a powernap, if you even have to explain it.

6.1.2 Not the Same Thing Again!—Dealing with Avoidance Behavior

Avoiding places, people, situations or thoughts that make you afraid is a successful strategy to stay away from what makes you afraid ... at least in the short term. Very short term.

If you are plagued by fear of many people, then it will first of all be better for you if you do not have to go to the next big company meeting. Not going there at first will result in the fear, the burden and the tension falling away. If you are plagued by the fear of darkness, then it will be better for you at first if you are at home before dark every day and can leave the light on there until the next morning.

It is also quite understandable that after one has made an existentially threatening experience, one does not want to get into such a situation again or one similar to it.

However, in the medium and long term, this avoidance behaviour will then increasingly become a problem in itself. Avoidance behaviour has the property of spreading. This process is called generalisation. By avoiding situations in the outside world that are associated with fear, or thoughts and feelings in the inside, the human brain learns that this coping strategy is quite successful, because there are the short-term successes in the form of fear reduction, etc. As a result, the human brain applies this avoidance behaviour to other situations in which there is fear. As a result, those affected increasingly avoid places, people, situations, thoughts and feelings.

In every situation in which something is avoided, the brain is also deprived of the experience of experiencing and learning from it that it can be mastered. This avoidance behaviour deprives the brain of the success experiences. The only thing that remains is the deep conviction that one can only fight for security through avoidance. At the end of an "avoidance career" is usually the social isolation and the fear as a permanent companion.

How can one deal with avoidance? What can one do against avoidance?

Do not avoid! This sounds very simple at first, but it is not.

At the beginning, an honest and open overview must be created of what one already avoids. As with the treatment of anxiety disorders, a hierarchy should be created with the things that scare one the most and whose avoidance causes the most suffering. Then a detailed plan should be created, with perhaps many intermediate steps, of how to face the fear and the avoidance behavior and reduce both of them successively. The individual intermediate steps should be chosen so that they always bring success experiences with them. Intermediate steps are also not set in stone and should be adapted according to the individual's current situation. Interim lows and setbacks are part of it. There may be moments from time to time when the fear was too great and it was still avoided. However, the avoidance behavior should become less and less from day to day, from week to week, from month to month.

In the end, it is also about developing a healthy and as objective as possible view of potential dangers: There are dangers in this world. At certain times of day, for example, one should rather avoid certain areas. It is not sensible to call such a healthy safety behavior into question, but it is about precisely analyzing and assessing situations for their danger.

One possible approach to reducing avoidance behavior could look like this:
- Creating an overview of the avoidance behavior so far.
  - What is avoided/avoided? (Situations? Places? People? Thoughts? Feelings?)
  - Since when is it avoided/avoided? Has the avoidance changed since then?
  - When is avoided/avoided?
  - How is avoided/avoided?
- Creating a hierarchy of what scares and what is avoided because of it.
- Creating a plan with intermediate steps to reduce avoidance behavior.
- Replacing avoidance behavior with security behavior.
- Plan for setbacks.
- After each non-avoidance, determine what will be changed next time to avoid even less.

In the individual situations in which one would like to avoid, one should proceed according to the principle of the 3 F. This simple strategy helps to avoid avoidance and to leave the fear behind.

The 3-F's for Avoidance Reduction and Anxiety Management
- **Focus it!**—Focus on the problem/fear.
  This is about becoming aware that certain things are avoided because certain situations are feared. It is about understanding what the problem is.

- **Face it!**—Be present to the problem/fear.
  Once it has been understood where the problem lies, it is about entering the situation. It is about not avoiding. This will inevitably lead to tension and fear increasing. Be aware of this. Do not distract yourself. This tension and fear will decrease on their own after a few minutes, at the latest after about 30 min. This decrease is due to biology. Be aware of this decrease too. This will teach your brain that nothing really bad is happening.
- **Fade it!**—Let go of the problem/fear.
  Every time you have endured a situation that you actually wanted to avoid; experienced that the tension and fear decrease, your brain learns this anew. In the medium and long term, this will result in the peaks of tension and fear becoming smaller and flatter. In the end, the situation that you used to avoid may only cause a slight discomfort in you.

6.1.3 Always under Pressure!—Dealing with Hyperarousal

Hyperarousal, also called hyperarousal, means a permanently inner tension or inner unrest. The body's own alarm system, the amygdala in the brain, is constantly looking for a potential danger. The affected people are very startled and need a long time to calm down after they are scared. Memory and concentration decline because a lot of brain capacity is used for this survival. Reading becomes more and more difficult because it becomes difficult to concentrate until the end of a page or even a sentence. And sleep is bad. Not only does it lead to painful nightmares through the re-experience, the affected people also do not come to rest.

The traumatization was a super-GAU for the body's own alarm system (amygdala). The alarm image of the trauma has been imprinted in the amygdala. This makes the sensitivity to the triggerability of the alarm reaction significantly increased.

This results in the fact that the affected people live with a very high basic tension level. But they are also more susceptible to stress from outside or inside. They have less buffer upwards and are thus faster at a stress limit.

Sleep is now one of the most dangerous factors for the alarm system. The amygdala works at full speed all day long to immediately recognize the slightest danger. In the evening, the alarm system should "agree" that the person enters a dark room, lies down, closes his eyes and sleeps. In this situation of sleep, the person is helplessly exposed to potential dangers. Therefore, the amygdala also rebels and prevents the affected person from sleeping. From the perspective of the amygdala, a sensible and successful strategy—from the perspective of the affected person, it is exhausting, exhausting.

The basic idea in dealing with overexcitement is to make the almond kernel calmer again. This is achieved by lowering the basic tension level and thus improving sleep, concentration and attention.

Strategies for reducing overexcitement are breathing exercises, imagination exercises, meditation, progressive muscle relaxation (PMR), autogenic training, yoga, mindfulness and many, many others. The goal of these strategies is to lower the basic tension level and allow better self-calming.

- **Breathing Exercises**

Breathing is what we always have with us. Breathing is life. And through the perception and control of our breath, we can directly influence our body, our thoughts and our emotions. Breathing is also the basis of many other relaxation methods, such as yoga or meditation.

Tich Nhat Hanh, a Vietnamese Buddhist monk and writer, once said:

> As we practice conscious breathing, our thinking slows down and we can experience real relaxation. Most of the time we think too much and mindful breathing helps us to be calm, relaxed and peaceful. It helps us to stop thinking so much and being obsessed with grief over the past and worries about the future. It helps us to get in touch with the life that is wonderful in the present moment.

The parasympathetic, which is part of the autonomic nervous system responsible for, among other things, rest and relaxation, can be activated by a simple trick. The overexcitement is mediated by the sympathetic, which is the other part of the autonomic nervous system responsible for, among other things, fight or flight. If you exhale a little longer than you inhale, you activate the parasympathetic. This in turn will lead to relaxation.

> **Breathing Exercise "One—One", "One—Out"**
> Take a comfortable sitting or standing position.
> Allow yourself to be completely focused on your breath for a few minutes.
> If you feel very tense, take two or three deep breaths to breathe out this tension.
> Now put your whole attention on your breath.
> Breathe in, say in your mind "one—one".
> Now breathe out a little longer than you inhaled and say in your mind "one—out".
> Breathe in again, say in your mind "two—one".
> Breathe out a little longer than you inhaled and say in your mind "two—out".
> Breathe in—"three—one".
> Breathe out a little longer—"three—out".
> "Four—one".
> "Four—out".
> Continue until you reach ten.

- **Imagination Exercises**

Imagination exercises play an important role in the treatment of a trauma-related disorder. Current research has now shown that imaginative processes trigger activity in similar brain areas as the actual action. So imagination is a great power, a power within. And that's where the reliving, the overexcitement, the horror of the trauma is.

A very important and actually indispensable imagination exercise in trauma therapy is the "inner safe place". In this imagination exercise, which was first described by Luise Reddemann, the central theme is safety. In the imagination, a place should be created, regardless of whether it exists or not, where people with PTSD feel safe. During the exercise, everything should be perceived at this place with all senses. Often it is necessary to develop and expand this place over a long period of time. Much of what initially seemed safe is not and must be removed or changed. In addition, it takes a lot of practice to achieve the full effect of the imagination exercise.

For this reason, the 3-3-3 rule should be applied to the imagination exercise—carry out the exercise 3 times a day for 3 min and do this for at least 33 days. Only then is it slowly ingrained. And only then can an assessment be made as to whether this imagination exercise helps or not.

The Inner Safe Place According to Luise Reddemann (Reddemann, 2007)

Take about 15 min for yourself during which you are uninterrupted as much as possible. Develop an image in your mind of a place where you feel absolutely safe, comfortable, and sheltered … This can be a place where you have been before. Maybe you remember a place that was special to you and had a healing effect on you … But it can also be a place that you imagine in your fantasy, that you read about once or dreamed of. In your imagination, anything is possible … It is a place that only you can enter and at most friendly, helpful beings that you summon or call. People should not have access to this place. Take your time and look for such a place … Maybe you see pictures … maybe you feel something … maybe you just think of such a place at first. Let whatever appear and accept it … If unpleasant images or thoughts should arise during your search for the safe inner place—which can happen once—then do not pay attention to them as much as possible and continue. Be assured that there is such a safe place for you and you just have to be patient for a while. It may be that the Searching for proximity is one thing, but it could also be that he is very far away somewhere in this world / in this universe … Please be aware that when searching for and designing your safe inner place, all conceivable aids are available to you, e.g. vehicles, tools, materials and even magical aids. If you feel that you have found a place where you feel comfortable and safe, then give it a name of your choice … Now check whether you are really completely safe there and feel comfortable. Look to see if you can make yourself comfortable there. It is important that you feel completely comfortable, safe and secure there. So please set up your safe inner place in such a way that this is possible. Take your time, imagine it all exactly and describe it to yourself in your mind … If you have found your safe inner place and designed it for your complete well-being and safety, sit down there for a while and please pay attention to how your body feels there, in this safe place. Take your time. What do you see?—What do you hear?—What do you smell?—What do you feel on your skin?—How are your muscles?—How is your breathing?—How is your stomach?—Does the temperature at your safe place meet your needs? Please take this very seriously so that you know how it feels to be in this safe place. Stay at your place for a moment and enjoy the feeling of well-being, safety and security that your place gives you … So that it is easier for you to return to your safe place in the future, agree with yourself now on a sign with which you can go to your safe place at any time. This can be a small body gesture that you often perform or a new small gesture. It would be good if you performed the gesture now and at the same time thought intensively about your safe place again … In this way you associate your safe place with this gesture in your imagination. Whenever you make this gesture in the future, you can go to your safe place and feel it. Please feel once again how good you feel in this safe place and then please come back into the room in which you are.

- **Autogenic Training**

Autogenic training is one of the best known relaxation methods in Europe. It was developed in the 1920s by the Berlin neurologist J. H. Schultz. He noticed that some of his patients, whom he treated with hypnosis, had taught themselves after a while to put themselves into a state that was very similar to hypnosis. In this state they were relaxed, calm and could perceive heaviness or warmth in their bodies.

The individual exercises of autogenic training are very simple and schematic. Certain formulas (e.g. "right arm heavy", "both legs warm" or "heart beats calmly and evenly") are spoken in the mind. At the same time, the focus is on body awareness.

> **Autogenes Training—"Heavy" Exercise**
> Take a comfortable standing, sitting or lying position.
> Breathe in and out two or three times. Close your eyes.
> Allow yourself to relax for a few minutes now.
> Tell yourself in your mind "very calm … very relaxed … the peace is deeper."
> Feel the peace in your body:
> Tell yourself in your mind now "The right arm is heavy … right arm heavy … right arm heavy."
> Take the weight in your right arm.
> Tell yourself in your mind now "The left arm is heavy … left arm heavy … left arm heavy."
> Take the weight in your left arm.
> Tell yourself in your mind now "Both arms are heavy … both arms heavy … both arms heavy."
> Take the weight in your arms.
> Tell yourself in your mind now "The shoulders are heavy … shoulders heavy … shoulders heavy."
> Take the weight in your shoulders.
> Tell yourself in your mind now "The body is heavy … body heavy … body heavy."
> Take the weight in your body.
> Tell yourself in your mind now "Heavy … Heavy … Heavy."
> Take the weight.
> Breathe in and out again two or three times. Open your eyes.
> Stretch.

- **Progressive Muscle Relaxation**

Edmund Jacobsen first described this relaxation technique in 1929. For this reason, it is often called Progressive Muscle Relaxation after Jacobsen.

In the exercises, different muscle groups are successively tense for a short time (approx. 5 to 10 s) while being aware of it. This tension is consciously perceived. After the time has elapsed, this muscle group is consciously relaxed again. This relaxation is consciously perceived again.

PMR Exercise

Breathe in and out two or three times deeply.
Focus your attention on your right hand and forearm. Make a fist, count to ten and breathe calmly.
When you reach ten, release the tension while exhaling.
Take the relaxation consciously for about a minute.
Focus your attention on your right upper arm and tense the muscles there, count to ten and breathe calmly.
When you reach ten, release the tension while exhaling.
Take the relaxation consciously for about a minute.
Focus your attention on your left hand and forearm. Make a fist, count to ten and breathe calmly.
When you reach ten, release the tension while exhaling.
Take the relaxation for about one minute consciously.
Focus your attention on your left upper arm and tense the muscles there, count to ten and breathe calmly.
When you arrive at ten, release the tension while exhaling
Take the relaxation for about one minute consciously.
Proceed with the following muscle groups according to this scheme:
- Forehead—frown
- Eyes—squint
- Lips—press lips together
- Shoulders—pull up to the ears
- right thigh
- right calf
- right foot
- left thigh
- left calf
- left foot

Breathe in and out two or three times deeply.

In addition to the described strategies, there are many, many more, the authors perhaps even unknown strategies for reducing the basic tension and overexcitement.

In addition, the principle of mindfulness should be considered here with the mindfulness exercises, which also leads to a reduction in the basic tension level.

6.1.4 When Half the Day is Missing!—Dealing with Dissociations

Dissociations often lead to different sized time gaps in memory. These time gaps are described as amnestic phases and those affected usually have no memory or only very vague and fragmented memories for this period of time. Through these memory gaps, those affected experience suffering. The dissociations restrict them in the design of their lives to a certain extent.

So how can you deal with dissociations and reduce them?

Dissociations are experienced by those affected and especially by those who experience a dissociation as a "spectator" as very dangerous, even life-threatening. A person is no longer responsive, may even have their eyes closed. The first measure is then often to call the emergency services. And if it is unclear whether it is a dissociation, this is also a very reasonable approach. However, if such situations occur more frequently, emergency services are no longer a solution. That is why it is important that those affected and their environment are conveyed and that they remind themselves again and again that dissociation is not life-threatening. The negative thing about dissociations is "only" that you don't learn anything new in them.

There are some strategies for dealing with dissociations and reducing them.

- **Recognize Triggers**

Dissociations are often caused by certain stimuli (triggers). These triggers can be very different stimuli from the outside or from within the affected person, a noise, a smell, or even a thought or a certain body experience. These triggers are often very typical for each affected person. Therefore, it should be worked on to identify these triggers, to name them and to remember them.

It is also important to mention that not everything that causes stress in an individual is a trigger. Every person is exposed to stressors and stimuli every day that cause stress and are experienced as unpleasant. Stimuli that cause stress in people are "stressors".

Triggers are, however, stimuli that cause a feeling of massive overstrain in the individual and he or she therefore presses the "dissociation button".

Every trigger is a stressor, but not every stressor is a trigger.

This should be considered when working on the triggers, otherwise an infinitely long list of stimuli will result, all of which are stressors, but only some of which are really triggers.

- **Dissociation Chain**

People affected by dissociations initially experience the onset of dissociations as sudden and "coming out of the blue". Dissociations do not start from one moment to the next. Most of the time, those affected go through a very typical sequence of forerunners. This sequence is called dissociation chain. Work should be done on this dissociation chain so that it becomes increasingly clear and obvious how dissociation occurs.

To improve understanding of the dissociation chain, it is advisable to analyze each dissociation in detail. This can be done using the following scheme:
– Before starting the analysis, those affected should first be fully present in the here and now and sufficiently stabilized after a dissociation.

6.1 · What Can I Do Myself—Strategies …

- Then the following questions should be answered:
  - What is the last thing you remember before the dissociation? (In what situation were you? What were you doing? Who else was there? Sounds? Smells? Conversations? Feelings? Thoughts? Body experience? …)
  - What is the last thing you remember before that?
  - What is the last thing you remember before that?
  - etc.

What those affected remember should be noted down. In addition, those affected should make it their business to pay attention to what they have worked out in the last dissociation analysis the next time they dissociate.

After the next dissociation, an analysis is again carried out according to the above points. Most of the time, the chain expands, as new insights arise from each dissociation analysis. Through this work, the dissociation chain grows successively.

The purpose of this dissociation chain is that those affected will very early on realize that there are signs of dissociation. If they recognize this, an early anti-dissociative approach is possible. The earlier intervention can take place, the better the chances that no dissociation will occur.

▪▪ Example of a Dissociation Chain
First there is a diffuse feeling of discomfort, then the legs feel strange and numb, then the voices of the people around sound muffled, then one only perceives the environment as if through cotton wool and then the dissociation occurs.

▪ Anti-Dissociative Strategies
There are very many different strategies in the fight against dissociations. One of them are skills.

Skills are sensory stimuli, strategies or techniques that help to reduce tension and to stay better in the here and now, that is, not to dissociate. Originally, skills were described and summarized by Marsha M. Linehan in the DBT therapy program she developed for sufferers of borderline personality disorder.

▪▪ Examples of Skills
- have an hedgehog ball in the hand
- consciously perceive the ground under the feet
- take a cold shower
- smell certain smells (the scent should have been chosen by the affected person in peace beforehand)
- listen to music
- look at beautiful pictures

▪ Other Strategies against Dissociations are
- 5-4-3-2-1-exercise: First find 5 blue, then 4 red, then 3 green, then 2 black, then 1 yellow object in the room.
- 100-minus-7-exercise: Subtract 7 from 100, then subtract 7 from the result, then subtract 7 from this result, etc.
- Say the alphabet backwards.

Dissociations can also be influenced by a conscious design of everyday life. The following points are important for this:
- drink enough fluid (at least 1.5 L per day); there is a direct connection between dissociation and low fluid intake
- eat well and enough
- do not consume drugs
- pay attention to regular and sufficient sleep
- move enough

Often the question arises as to how colleagues, relatives, friends and family should deal with dissociations. First of all, it is important that these people receive enough information so that they can understand what is happening. In addition, they should understand that a dissociation is not a dangerous situation.

When dealing with dissociative people, the following tips can be given:
- address the person, but do not touch
- radiate calm
- tell the person where he is and who you are
- ask the person to come to the here and now
- clap your hands carefully
- 5-4-3-2-1 exercise: The person should first name 5 blue, then 4 red, then 3 green, then 2 black, then 1 yellow object in the room
- if the person is already back in the here and now, motivate him to apply the skills
- humor! Humor activates brain regions responsible for mentalization and therefore reorients very well.

6.1.5 When the Mind Falls into the Trap!—The 10 Most Important Cognitive PTSD Traps

Traumatic experiences often leave those affected with distorted thoughts about the trauma and themselves, especially in terms of their behavior in the traumatic situation. These thoughts in turn lead to distorted and dysfunctional basic assumptions about themselves, the world, and other people. In the end, these thoughts often result in the affected people assigning themselves blame. In behavioral therapy, the identification, naming, analysis, and correction of such cognitions is worked on very specifically.

These, typical cognitive traps for people with PTSD (according to Kubany, 1997) are:
- **The "gut feeling" trap:**
  The "bad gut feeling" that was experienced before the traumatic situation is retrospectively seen as proof that one should have seen it coming. The many thousands of times that one has such a feeling, and then nothing happens, are not taken into account in the considerations.
  Be the rational manager: What's the point of looking back? Can you change what happened? No. Look ahead and optimize today's and future actions. No one will ever know what would have happened if you had listened to your gut

feeling and a different action had taken place. Because it is just a gut feeling and not an objective proof.

- **The Knowledge Trap:**
  In the retrospective assessment of the traumatic situation, the affected person attributes to themselves that they should have known what would happen because there were signs of it, even though this is not the case.
  It is impossible to know and predict everything that will happen. Retrospective assessments often involve seeing signs that were not actually present in the situation itself. Even the best manager has to admit that he cannot always know what will happen.

- **The Prevention Trap:**
  The affected person attributes to themselves that they could have prevented what happened, even though this is not objectively the case.
  No matter how much public influence or power you have at your disposal, no matter how much experience you have gathered, some things just happen. And you have no influence on them, you cannot prevent them. No matter how close it may have been or how strong or weak you may have been. Nobody can know whether you really had a chance to intervene at all.

- **The causation trap:**
  Could the event have been objectively prevented in any way? This thought includes the fact that the affected persons did not do this. It does not mean that they also caused the event.
  Even if there had really been a way to prevent the traumatic event, that does not mean that it could have been prevented by the person affected.

- **The guilt trap:**
  In some situations, a person has a responsibility for something and has to make decisions within the framework of this responsibility. It can always happen that something traumatic happens when a decision is made. Having responsibility for a situation does not mean that one is also to blame for it.
  In particular, in leadership positions you carry the burden of responsibility. In most cases you make the right decisions objectively. But everyone who has responsibility can also make wrong decisions or has to make decisions whose effects are still unpredictable at the time of the decision or even cause suffering in parts. It would be a violation of your responsibility not to decide. You have decided and it may have caused suffering. This does not automatically make the event your fault.

- **The Monocausal Fallacy:**
  The traumatic situation, like any situation in life, had several causes. However, those affected retrospectively isolate one cause. A monocausal explanation is very convenient for the human mind because it is simple, but it does not correspond to reality.
  Things that happen rarely have only one cause. As a manager, you are aware of this. Complex relationships have consequences. Simple explanation patterns are always suspicious. Do not fall for it yourself.

- **The "no chance" trap:**
  Those affected do not see retrospectively that all decision options that existed in the traumatic situation had negative aspects. Sometimes only one decision is possible for the least bad option.

Especially in leadership positions it is your task to decide. Sometimes there is no decision that can be considered good objectively, because every option has negative consequences. But then to decide anyway and to make the least bad decision is a strength.

- **The "Cherries in Neighbor's Garden" trap:**
In the traumatic situation, the affected persons made decisions. Perhaps they could have made others. Retrospectively, the non-decisions are seen as those that could have prevented the trauma, without this being the case.

- **The intentions trap:**
The affected persons do not judge their actions before and in the traumatic situation from the standpoint of the actual action intention, but from that of the result. They do not ask, "What did I want to achieve?", But "What did I achieve?" And set it equal.
Hindsight is always wiser. A "clichéd phrase", but it is correct in content. You cannot base your assessment of what has happened on the information that is available to you then after an event. It is not about what actually happened, but what was the state of affairs before the event and what you might have done to achieve which goal. This cannot be reinterpreted with the knowledge afterwards. Your actual intention at the time of the decision made is relevant.

- **The "supernatural forces" trap:**
Affected people retrospectively overestimate their knowledge (a lot of knowledge, insights, judgments come later and are created through long consideration, which was not possible in the traumatic situation) and their ability to act in the traumatic situation. In addition, physiological reactions of the body are not accepted.
In addition, traumatic situations are characterized by the fact that they fall out of the normal experience. They therefore represent an exceptionally high burden for those affected. This burden is often not taken into account in the assessment of one's own actions by those affected. If I have to flee from a burning house, I will not make great deliberations.
As a manager or experienced person in the public eye, you are subject to special requirements. But don't make them superhuman either. To a certain extent, you can better assess than others, especially in such extraordinary stress situations. But not so much more that you would have the strength to do superhuman things. There are many things that no human being can influence. No matter how well trained or trained he is. Some things are just coincidence, luck or misfortune. Be aware of this. You can't do everything, even if you want to or it would have been right and good. It is simply impossible. You can only make the best of what is possible. As a good manager, you know your possibilities and limits. Don't question yourself afterwards. Trust yourself. As always, see the big picture, the big picture.

Such cognitive traps should be identified, named and processed during psychotherapy in order to achieve a correction.

6.1.6 Thought Carousel!—Dealing with Thought Circles

Thought circles and brooding is a common symptom of PTSD and usually manifests itself in the evening, when those affected are in bed and actually want to sleep. In the head, the same thoughts are then gone through over and over again. Horrible scenarios are drawn, everything seems much worse, bigger, more threatening.

Thought circles and brooding have a lot, but no end and no solution. That's what makes brooding: a continuous thinking about problems and situations without any solution or insight.

In dealing with brooding, the thought stop technique has proven itself. For this it is first of all necessary that those affected by brooding recognize the situation in which they brood.

> Point 1 is therefore the recognition that one is brooding.

If this is recognized, a decision must be made: Should one continue to brood or not? If you decide against brooding, you should also formulate it in your thoughts. You can say to yourself: "I'm now stopping to brood!" In addition, you can imagine a stop sign that signals to you the decision to stop brooding.

> Point 2 is therefore the decision not to brood anymore.

But the human mind wants to be busy. For this reason, it is important to turn to something else after the anti-brooding decision, e.g. reading, listening to music, making tea.

> Point 3 is therefore to consciously turn to another activity than brooding.

During the first few times, the worrying thoughts will come back after a few seconds. Then it is necessary to decide against it again and to turn to something else.

> Point 4 is therefore to decide against worrying again and again.

The secret of a successful thought-stopping technique is that one has decided against worrying again and again, as the worrying came back.

A little trick is the worry book. If the same worrying thoughts keep coming back, you can take a little notebook or a sheet and write down what you are worrying about. If it is then written down, you can consciously agree a date with yourself for the next day, at which you think or worry about this topic for a certain period of time (approx. 15 min). By writing down and postponing to another date, it is often possible to solve these thoughts better.

6.1.7 When Fears Determine Life!—Dealing with Fears

Fears play an important role in the lives of people with PTSD. They often determine large parts of life. In addition, the fears contribute to avoidance behavior. Therefore, one can deal with the fears similarly to avoidance behavior.

One possible approach could look like this:

- Creating an overview of what causes fear
    - What causes fear? (Situations? Places? People? Thoughts? Feelings?)
    - Since when has this been a fear? Has the fear changed since then?
    - When does the fear come?
    - How is the fear experienced?
- Creating a fear hierarchy
- Creating a plan with intermediate steps for exposure to fears
- Plan for setbacks

In the individual situations in which one experiences fear, one should deal with this fear according to the principle of the "3 F".

The 3-F's for avoidance reduction and anxiety management (Matten & Pausch, 2017):
- **Focus it!**—Focus on the anxiety.
    This is about becoming aware that certain things cause anxiety. It is about understanding what this anxiety is about.
- **Face it!**—Be aware of the anxiety.
    Once you have understood where the anxiety lies, it is about getting into the situation. It is about not avoiding it. This will inevitably lead to tension and anxiety increasing. Be aware of this consciously. Do not distract yourself. This tension and anxiety will decrease again after a few minutes, at the latest after about 30 min. This decrease is due to biology. Be aware of this decrease consciously. This will teach your brain that nothing really bad happens.
- **Fade it!**—Let go of the anxiety.
    Every time you have endured a situation that you wanted to avoid, experienced that the tension and anxiety decrease, your brain learns this again. In the medium and long term, this will result in the peaks of tension and anxiety becoming smaller and flatter. In the end, the situation that you used to avoid may only cause a slight discomfort in you.

Nobody has to allow fear, or even the fear of fear, to determine their life. The first step in dealing with one's own fear and one's own fear symptoms is a good understanding of fear and the situations in which fear comes, as well as learning how to react to it individually in the best way possible. Fear and trauma are closely interwoven. Sometimes an anxiety disorder has to do with traumatic experiences or

PTSD. PTSD is usually associated with fears. Thus, a constructive approach to fear, which can be learned, plays a significant role in dealing with PTSD.

Ask yourself the "why" question and see it as the key to a successful start on the road to solving fear. Understanding and awareness help in dealing with fear both in the acute phase and in the long-term work on it. You can do this alone or with support from outside. If you accept support from outside, get professional help. Depending on the social or professional situation, this can be a personal coach, a psychiatrist or a psychologist, a psychotherapist or a general practitioner. At this point, no compromises should be made, at least not of a qualitative nature. Trust yourself and your body. And at the same time, always clarify any possible medical physical causes of your fear and its symptoms. Fear is a force. Use it as an opportunity, don't let it drive you, but tame it and don't lose sight of the goal: In the end you will be stronger than before and have grown significantly. objectively speaking, you usually don't have any other choice: You have to deal with your fear and find solutions. So you can do this right away, targeted and effectively in implementation.

Nobody can say that it is easy to deal with fear. In the phase of fear, every talk about fear and any kind of dealing with it seems ridiculous and unrealistic. But there are also phases between fear. It is particularly important then to have as sober a purely factual realistic view as possible. Even if the level of fear remains constant and the fear of fear torments: In this time one can become active well. It doesn't help to avoid.

Nobody is a single case. There are many affected people in all social and economic classes and at all levels of employment: from the housewife and mother or the househusband and father involved in a family, to the single person, employees or unemployed people, to people in professional leadership positions and public figures.

6.1.8 What to Do about Pain?

The International Association for the Study of Pain (IASP) defines pain as "an unpleasant sensory and emotional experience associated with actual or potential tissue damage or described in terms of such damage."

Pain can occur as acute pain and then usually has mainly physical causes. Pain has a clear warning function. The corresponding treatment is then also a physical treatment.

To give an example: A broken arm hurts and warns the affected person that something is wrong with the arm. The treatment of this pain is a physical one, namely an operation or a plaster.

However, it may also be that pain is shown chronically, that is, over a longer period of time (longer than 3 months). Often, the physical component is then lower. The perception and processing of pain is strongly linked to the mental state. In chronic pain, physical examinations often do not find clear causes. In chronic pain, the soul can make the body suffer. The psyche has no organ and therefore makes other organs suffer on its behalf.

Everyone has a pain threshold, from which he perceives a pain. This threshold depends on how strong, balanced, satisfied and relaxed he is. So this threshold fluctuates not only from individual to individual, but also from moment to moment. Stress, strain, depression, sleep deficit, etc. lead to the fact that this threshold decreases. As a result, those affected perceive even less pain than if the threshold were higher.

In addition, pain in PTSD sufferers can be memory pain, that is, intrusions.

The management of chronic pain is often very difficult and poses a problem that requires the cooperation of many medical disciplines.

For those affected, it is important to recognize the connection between pain threshold and load. Because at this point an intervention can take place. Any strategy that leads to reduced stress, less load, the individual more balanced, will lead to the fact that the pain threshold rises and thus less pain is perceived.

In addition, one should work with people suffering from chronic pain and PTSD on the control of attention focus. Even if there is pain, one should move one's attention away from it. The less you focus the pain in the focus of attention, the less it will be perceived.

In the treatment of chronic pain and PTSD, a reasonable diagnostics, anamnesis and treatment planning, in cooperation with pain specialists, is necessary. Under certain circumstances, a pure treatment with specialists for chronic pain is necessary.

6.1.9 When the Night Becomes Day!—Dealing with Sleep Disorders

On average, a person spends one third of his life sleeping. With nothing else, man spends more time dreaming. In sleep various sleep phases are traversed. These sleep phases are distributed differently throughout the night. Sleep is very important for our brain in terms of learning new things.

But sleep also poses a danger to our body and our psyche, because then the ability to respond to a potential danger is very low. Therefore, sleep disorders often occur in PTSD sufferers. The overexcitement and the fear are often too great to find sleep. The rumination is too powerful for the mind to find peace. And the fear of the next nightmare is too great.

What prevents restful sleep are therefore many different factors that need to be addressed individually and extra. Nevertheless, there are basic rules on how to improve your sleep. The term sleep hygiene often falls in this context. This refers to certain behaviors that generally contribute to the fact that sleep improves.

Therefore, pay attention to these points when you have difficulty falling asleep or staying asleep:
- Keep to regular times for going to bed and getting up.
- Don't sleep during the day, even if you're very tired.
- Only use the bed for sleeping.
- Don't go to bed either hungry or stuffed.
- Pay attention to your consumption of nicotine, caffeine, and alcohol. All three substances have a significant effect on sleep.
- No physical or mental overexertion about 3 h before going to bed.

- If you can't sleep, don't stay in bed awake for longer than 30 min. Get up, do something calming, and try to sleep again later.
- Make sure you feel safe and secure in your bedroom and bed.
- Create a bedtime routine.
- Avoid sleeping pills.

6.1.10 When Addiction has You in its Grip!—Dealing with Addiction

If a PTBS is accompanied by a comorbid addiction, it is important to also carry out a precise diagnosis of the addiction, including any possible physical consequences. It must be clarified which addiction is present. Sometimes there are also several addictions. If there is already a physical symptom that requires immediate medical treatment, this must be initiated.

If this is not necessary, or completed, the next step is a precise treatment planning. In this context, it must be clarified which of the two diseases, PTBS or addiction, has priority. In most cases, a physical detoxification treatment is first necessary in the case of a comorbid addiction. If this is successfully completed, it must be clarified whether a withdrawal treatment must be immediately connected or whether a stabilization phase is better at first. Although a combination would be a good idea, there are no specialized facilities for this in Germany.

After clarification and implementation of the withdrawal and sufficient stabilization, it must be determined when sufficient stability for a confrontation treatment is given.

During the confrontation treatment, the addiction behavior should continue to be monitored. Under the strain of a confrontation, it can happen that the addiction to the drug becomes stronger again. If this is the case, countermeasures must be taken and the confrontation may be paused.

After successful completion of the confrontation treatment, the connection to a self-help group should continue during the reorientation phase.

Addiction is a very taboo and stigmatized topic. The admission of an addiction is usually seen as a weakness and experienced. That is why it is important to make it clear again and again that addiction is also a disease and can be treated well—but only if the affected persons also seek treatment.

Therefore, the following is important for those affected:

> If you notice that you meet some of the above-mentioned criteria for addiction, be brave and get help. Go to your GP, a psychiatrist, an addiction counseling, a self-help group.

6.2 Resources

PTSD is characterized by the fact that those affected feel helpless, unable, deficient, weak. Therefore, it is important to also look at the resources of the respective person.

> **Resources**
>
> The word "resources" comes from the French (source for "source"). This refers to strengths, abilities, helpfulness and positives in a person and in his life.

Sometimes these resources, which every person has, are overlaid or lost through the traumatization and one has to search for them again. In order to achieve this, a resource analysis is very helpful. It is best to keep your resources in writing so that there is always the opportunity to fall back on them if everything seems hopeless again and you are yourself "incapable".

❓ Resource Analysis / Resource Diagram—Answer the Following Questions, Preferably in Writing
- What used to make you happy?
- What could you always do especially well?
- What did you like to do most of the time as a child/teenager?
- When were you always asked for advice? What was it about?
- Which academic, extracurricular, and professional achievements have you made?
- What was your favorite subject in school?
- What else would you like to achieve professionally?
- What else would you like to achieve outside of work? Travel? Learn a new language?
- What were your hobbies?
- When and where can you relax?
- Who are the most important people in your life?
- What connects you to these people?
- What were the 5 most beautiful moments in your life?
- Is there a belief in your life?

Look at what you have noted and realize what treasures you already have in your life, what strengths you already have.

Whenever you don't feel well, look at these notes.

6.3 General Basics of Trauma Therapy

Before the treatment of those affected by PTSD can begin, it is essential that a sound and comprehensive diagnosis is carried out. Before treatment begins, it must be clear what the actual problems are, that is, which specific diagnoses are present. In addition, it is important to pay attention to which comorbidities exist, because they must be included in a reasonable treatment plan. As part of such a diagnostic phase, it is very often necessary for those affected to fill out certain diagnosis questionnaires.

In the second step, it must be discussed with those affected in a clear and as concrete as possible what the individual goals of the therapy are. These goals must be the goals of those affected and not the ambitious goals of a therapist.

The therapy goals should be SMART. This acronym has become established in project management and helps to define goals as clearly as possible.

6.3 · General Basics of Trauma Therapy

> **SMART**
>
> The word "SMART" stands for **S**pecific, **M**easurable, **A**ccepted, **R**ealistic and **T**ime Bound (dt. **S**pezifisch, **M**essbar, **A**kzeptiert, **R**ealistisch, **T**erminiert).

With this method, the therapy goals can be formulated so that there are also success experiences during the treatment, for client / in and therapist / in.

If the diagnosis is clear and the therapy goals are formulated, they should be worked on.

When it comes to therapy goals and therapeutic interventions, a distinction must be made between those affected by a "simple" PTSD and those affected by a complex PTSD.

Both are divided into 3 parts: stabilization first, then confrontation and finally reorientation.

People with a "simple" PTSD often bring greater stability and better affect regulation into therapy, so that the first phase, the stabilization phase, can be shorter than with a complex PTSD. For those affected by a complex trauma disorder, the priority is to improve or establish their stability and to achieve an improvement in the regulation of affects. In addition, comorbidities must be treated in this first phase. This phase of treatment can last from a few weeks to a few years.

In the second part of the treatment, which one only enters when sufficient stability and affect regulation is achieved, it is about the trauma exposure or the trauma synthesis. Here, the person affected turns, accompanied by the therapist, again to the trauma. Through this re-engagement and the activation of the then experience, an integration of this trauma network can come about. The then faulty storage can be healed in this way, so to speak. In the context of confrontation treatment, there are different therapy methods that can be used.

In the third and final part of the therapy, the focus is on the new or reorientation. Here it is about planning the time after the therapy. It is often about very concrete questions, but also about questions about the meaning of what has happened to the person concerned.

Frederick Kanfer, a psychology professor at the University of Illinois, has divided the course of a psychotherapy into 7 phases (Kanfer et al., 2006):
1. Initial phase
2. Building motivation for change and selecting change areas
3. Behavioral analysis with description of the problem and the conditions for maintaining the problem
4. Clarifying and agreeing on goals in psychotherapy
5. Planning, selection and implementation of special methods for achieving goals
6. Assessment of therapeutic progress
7. Final phase with completion of psychotherapy

When transferring these 7 phases to the 3-phase trauma therapy, phases 1 to 4 would fall into the stabilization phase. Phases 5 and 6 take place in both the stabilization and confrontation and reorientation phases. Ultimately, phase 7 will take place in the reorientation phase.

6.4 Behavioral, Psychodynamic and Trauma-Specific Approaches

In trauma therapy, a cross-school understanding of the disorder is very common. If possible, various helpful strategies from different therapy schools will be used. So Louise Reddemann brought together a psychodynamic and a hypnotherapeutic approach. Nevertheless, in the different therapy directions, their own PTBS therapy procedures have been established.

The following methods have established themselves in cognitive behavioral therapy:
- prolonged exposure according to Foa
- trauma-focused cognitive behavioral therapy according to Ehlers and Clark
- cognitive processing therapy according to Resick
- **I**magery **R**escripting and **R**eprocessing **T**herapy (IRRT) according to Smucker

The following methods have been developed from the field of psychodynamic psychotherapy (i.e. depth psychological-based psychotherapy and psychoanalysis):
- **P**sychodynamic **I**maginative **T**rauma-**T**herapie (PITT) by Reddemann
- Psychodynamic trauma therapy by Horrowitz

In addition, there are methods that were not developed directly from a therapy school, but specifically for the treatment of PTSD. The most prominent of these is the Eye Movement Desensitization and Reprocessing (EMDR) developed by Francine Shapiro and the Narrative Exposure Therapy (NET).

The currently best evaluated therapy methods, which are considered the most promising, are trauma-focused cognitive behavioral therapy and EMDR.

The following will briefly discuss trauma-focused cognitive behavioral therapy and prolonged exposure, as these are two of the most important and promising methods. Afterwards, a closer look will be taken at confrontation methods. In doing so, the PITT, EMDR, IRRT and NET will also be briefly mentioned.

- **Trauma-Focused Cognitive Behavioral Therapy According to Ehlers and Clark**

The treatment developed by Ehlers and Clark includes the following points:
- With those affected, an individual model of disorder, illness and healing is worked out
- The affected persons receive all important information about the illness, incl. Symptom onset, symptom maintenance (psychoeducation)
- Learning of imagination methods for the imaginative reliving of the trauma (exposure in imagination)
- Identification and discrimination of the triggers of intrusions
- Exposure treatment
- Cognitive restructuring
- The behaviors that maintain the symptoms are identified and modified with cognitive strategies
- Working on the prevention of relapse

In addition, the focus is on the fact that those affected experience self-efficacy again, that is, they gain control over inner experience and outer behavior.

6.4 · Behavioral, Psychodynamic and Trauma-Specific Approaches

- **Prolonged Exposure According to Foa (2007)**

In this procedure, PTSD is viewed as an anxiety disorder. The individual therapy phases are briefly mentioned below.
- Creating the therapy plan and explaining the therapy process
- Hierarchy of the fear-related situation
- Exposure with the memories of the trauma in the imagination with a description of the memory in the present tense. An audio file is created from this part of the therapy, which the affected persons should listen to several times until the next session. In this way, it should be possible to experience a decrease in stress from one time to the next
- Exposure with feared situations or objects in reality

6.4.1 Stabilization Phase

As mentioned above, the first phase of trauma treatment is stabilization. The goal of this treatment phase is to achieve sufficient affect regulation and sufficient safety and stability in the lives of those affected. The treatment of comorbidities also falls into the stabilization phase. Under certain conditions, it is necessary that only the treatment of a comorbidity is carried out first, e.g. when it is necessary to make a withdrawal and detoxification treatment in the case of an addiction. The exact plan of treatment, including any preceding treatments, should take place after extensive professional consultation and in collaboration with a trauma therapist or trauma therapist.

Many different strategies, measures and interventions are used in the context of stabilization treatment. Some, from the perspective of the authors, are important. When selecting the following points, it was also a criterion whether a first implementation attempt was possible without therapeutic guidance.

Mindfulness and Level of Tension

In the Buddhist, especially Zen Buddhist, teaching and meditation, the principle of mindfulness has been a central element for over 2500 years.

> **Mindfulness**
>
> Mindfulness is the intention to experience the present moment consciously and to break out of automatic or purely mechanical behavior in order to be present in one's own life, not fruitlessly thinking into an uncertain future or clinging to an unpleasant past. The present moment is neither rejected nor idealized. Consequences are taken into account. A distinction is made between usefulness and harmfulness. One goes with the changing life without attachment.
>
> Mindfulness is a clear state of consciousness that is exclusively in the here and now. The thought "yesterday is gone, tomorrow is not yet here" is to lead to the awareness of the moment.

This form of awareness in the moment was introduced into Western psychotherapy by Jon Kabat-Zinn, who developed a systematic program for stress management through mindfulness. Later, American psychology professor Marsha Linehan developed a treatment manual for sufferers of borderline personality disorder, which includes mindfulness as a central principle. Meanwhile, mindfulness is an important part of the treatment of many mental disorders.

Every person has a certain tension in every situation. This tension level can be rated, for example, on a scale of 0% to 100%. Here 0% means no tension at all, and 100% means that the maximum conceivable tension is perceived. Every person can actively influence his or her own tension level. The first step is to become aware of where you are on the tension scale from 0% to 100%. To reduce tension, there are different possibilities, relaxation techniques, imagination exercises, or mindfulness.

The goal of mindfulness is to reduce suffering and increase joy, to increase control over one's own mind, and to experience reality as it is.

There is a distinction between inner and outer mindfulness.

Inner mindfulness means that a person's entire attention is directed inward and it is about precisely perceiving what is happening physically, emotionally, and cognitively within oneself.

Outer mindfulness, on the other hand, means that the focus of attention is directed outward and one perceives everything very precisely with one's senses.

M. Linehan divided mindfulness into being and how skills:

"What Skills" or the Question: What Am I Doing?
- **Perceive:** Perceive my outside through my senses—outer mindfulness. Give my thoughts, feelings, and bodily sensations space—inner mindfulness
- **Describe:** Find words for what my senses perceive—outer mindfulness. Find words for what is happening inside of me—inner mindfulness
- **Participate:** Be fully present, without distraction, whether in the outside or in the inside

"How-Skills" or the Question: How Do I Do It?
- **Non-evaluative:** Reality is as it is, and there are reasons for it. (Here the Buddhist principle of cause and effect is shown). Because things are as they are and there are reasons for it, it makes no sense to make a distinction between good and bad.
  Non-evaluative does not mean that one likes everything, but the recognition of the actual situation as it is in order then to decide which consequences arise from it for oneself.
- **Concentrated:** This is about staying focused and recognizing and stopping distractions.
- **Effective:** "Play the game effectively!"—The goal and the purpose of one's own actions should not be lost sight of.

In addition, M. Linehan described radical acceptance and the benevolent self (wise mind) as part of mindfulness.

> **Radical Acceptance**
>
> This means an inner accepting attitude towards external circumstances and feelings that cannot be changed. Through this attitude, reality is neither rejected nor fought, neither mentally nor real.

» Radical acceptance is the only way out of hell—it means giving up the fight against reality. Acceptance is the way that turns unbearable suffering into tolerable pain. Marsha Linehan

Mindfulness is a principle that can be excellently integrated into everyday life. Already in the morning after getting up, you can be fully present in the here and now and perceive it with all your senses while brushing your teeth.

Here are 2 examples of **mindfulness exercises**:

Walking Meditation

Dedicate your full attention to the process of walking while you are walking. First, stay still for a moment and try to feel your soles and what you perceive above them with full awareness. Notice how you are deeply rooted in the ground below you. To do this, you may first shift your weight slightly to your heels, then slightly forward to your toes. Make sure your shoulders are loose. Take three deep breaths in and out to get rid of any initial tension. Then let your breath flow freely. Take a step forward, lift your foot up, put it in front of your body with the heel and roll forward to the toes. Feel every perception in your foot and on your soles. Now take the other foot. Lift it up again, put it in front of your body with the heel and roll forward to the toes. Again, take notice of every little perception.

It is best to do this exercise barefoot.

Body Scan Meditation (Abridged from Segal et al., 2008)

Lie down and make yourself comfortable. Take a few moments and take contact with the movements of your breath and the sensations in your body. If you are ready, focus your attention on the sensations in your body, especially the sensations of touch and pressure, where your body is in contact with the mat. Allow yourself to let go with each exhalation and sink a little deeper into the ground. Now focus your attention on the physical sensations in the lower abdomen. As you inhale and exhale, you become aware of the changing patterns of sensations in the abdominal wall. Take a few minutes to feel these sensations as you continue to inhale and exhale. Once you have established a connection with the sensations in the abdomen, let the focus of your attention wander down the left leg and into the left foot, and to the toes of the left foot. Alternately focus on each individual toe of the left foot and bring gentle interest as you explore the quality of the sensations you find there; perhaps you feel the contact between your toes, a tickling, warmth, or no particular sensation. If you are ready, you can Inhale and imagine or feel how the breath enters the lungs and then descends into the abdominal cavity, down into the left leg, into the left foot, and to the toes of the left foot. Exhaling, you can feel or imagine how the breath comes back up the whole way, into the foot, into the leg, into the abdominal cavity, up through the chest and out through the nose. Do this for a few breaths, as best you can, breathing all the way down into the toes and back out again. It may be difficult at first to get a sense for this—just practice this "inhaling" as best you can and be playful with it. When you're ready, on the exhale let go of the attention on your toes and direct it towards the sensations in your left foot sole—bring your gentle, interested attention to the ball of the foot, the arch, the heel. Experiment with "breathing into" the sensations—be aware of the breath in the background as you explore the sensations in the lower part of the foot in the foreground. Now allow your awareness to expand to the rest of the foot—to the ankle, the top of the foot, and up to the bones and joints. Then take a slightly deeper breath and direct the breath to the whole left foot. And asbreathe out, let go of the breath, and also let go of the foot completely and allow the focus of your attention to move to the lower area of the left leg—to the calf, the shin, the knee, etc., one after the other. Continue to bring the physical sensations in each area of the rest of the body in turn your attention—to the upper area of the left leg, to the right toes, to the right foot, to the right leg, to the hip area, to the back, to the stomach area, to the chest, to the fingers, to the hands, to the arms, to the shoulders, to the neck, to the head and to the face. Bring the present physical sensations in each area as well as you can the same level of attention and gentle interest. If you become aware of tension or other intense sensations in a particular area of the body, you can "breathe into" it—by using the inhalation gently to direct your attention directly to these sensations and exhale the feeling to dissolve or release. After you have "scanned" the whole body in this way, spend a few minutes becoming aware of your body sensation as a whole. The breath flows freely through the body in and out. If you find that you are getting sleepy, you may find it helpful to support your head with a pillow, open your eyes, or do the exercise sitting instead of lying down.

Distancing Techniques

As part of trauma therapy, especially when it comes to a confrontation treatment, but also in everyday life, it is important that those affected by PTSD are given behaviors and strategies with which they can distance themselves from intrusive inner material and its effects on the individual, such as flashbacks, dissociations, rumination, pain.

There are a large number of strategies and techniques for this. Some of them have already been listed above. A small overview will be given here, knowing full well that this can only be a small selection.

> **Techniques for Distancing**
> — Focus attention on the here and now
>   – 3-2-1-exercise
>   – 100-minus-7-exercise
>   – Alphabet-exercise
> — Know triggers and dissociation / flashback chain
> — Skills

- Mindfulness exercises
- Breathing exercises and meditation
- Imagination exercise
  - inner safe place
  - vault exercise
- Relaxation techniques
  - Autogenic training
  - PMR
- Screen exercise
- Reality check

6.4.2 Confrontation Phase

In order to enter the confrontation phase, it is necessary that those affected have achieved sufficient stability. This means that there has been no serious self-injurious behavior, attempted suicide, high-risk behavior, or serious problems with foreign aggressiveness in the last four months. In addition, no confrontation treatment should be carried out if an acute psychosis is present. Caution should also be exercised with a confrontation treatment if there is an acute substance abuse or unstable psychosocial or physical situations (AWMF-S3-Guidelines Posttraumatic Stress Disorder, 2001).

In the confrontation phase of trauma therapy, those affected turn to the traumatic experiences again in therapeutic accompaniment. This means that the memories of what happened, as well as the feelings, thoughts and body reactions in the situation at that time and today when looking at the memories are activated again. This activation of the trauma network leads to the fact that it becomes "manageable", the faulty storage is canceled and the here-and-now memory becomes a there-and-then memory. With here-and-now memory is meant that the affected do not experience the memories as such, but remember the past event as if it were happening again in the here and now. Through the confrontation this can be turned into a there-and-then memory. The affected therefore remember that in the "there and then" this or that happened. The re-experience becomes a memory. The trauma is stored where it happened: in the past.

6.4.3 Reorientation Phase

After the completion of the confrontation treatment, the cause of PTSD is, so to speak, remedied. The intrusions have subsided, the nightmares of the trauma are only a memory. Those affected feel how peace and security return to their lives.

And yet there are questions, challenges that need to be accompanied therapeutically. In this part of trauma therapy, on the one hand, it is necessary to take another look back, to weave the trauma, the trauma-related disorder and the treatment into one's own biography. Here, questions of meaning are often asked. And it is about evaluating what has been achieved and accomplished. On the other hand, this phase of therapy is also about looking to the future. What's next? What are the next steps in life? And what are the next goals?

Finally, in this phase of treatment, it is about ending the therapy. Those affected have the task of gradually withdrawing from the therapeutic relationship, which in the renewed focus on the trauma has given stability and security.

6.5 Confrontation Procedures

6.5.1 EMDR

The treatment technique EMDR was developed by the US psychologist Francine Shapiro in the 1980s and 1990s for the treatment of trauma-related disorders.

> **EMDR**
>
> EMDR is an acronym that stands for **E**ye **M**ovement **D**esensitization and **R**eprocessing, which can be translated as "desensitization and processing through eye movement".

In 2006, the Scientific Advisory Board for Psychotherapy recognized EMDR as a scientifically based psychotherapy method. In recent years and decades, numerous scientific studies have confirmed the effectiveness of this therapy.

Trauma processing using EMDR takes place on 4 levels. These levels are:
1. visual level
2. cognitive level (thoughts)
3. emotional level (feelings)
4. Body and behavior

The procedure in EMDR is carried out according to the EMDR protocol (Shapiro, 2013), which includes 8 phases. Some of these phases include general treatment phases of the overall therapy plan.

The 8 phases are as follows:
1. Anamnesis and treatment planning
   This includes the collection of the exact medical and trauma history, biography, as well as diagnostics, as well as the collection of resources.
2. Preparation and stabilization
   In this phase, the theory of EMDR is explained and work is done on sufficient stability and affect regulation.
3. Assessment of the trauma
   The selected traumatic memory is worked on in relation to the 4 levels. First, an image is worked out which represents the worst moment of the memory. Then the thoughts of the person concerned in this traumatic situation (negative cognition; e.g. "I'm dying now!") and a desired target thought (positive cognition; e.g. "I survived!") are worked out. In relation to the target thought, it is determined

6.5 · Confrontation Procedures

how congruent this already feels for the person concerned on a scale from 1 ("does not match at all") to 7 ("completely congruent") (Validity of Cognition, VoC). Furthermore, the feelings that arise when looking at the memory are named and the current degree of stress (Subjective Units of Discomfort, SUD) is set on a scale from 0 (no stress) to 10 (maximum conceivable stress). Finally, the body sensations that occur when contacting the traumatic memory are recorded. Through this procedure of trauma assessment, the trauma network is reactivated and thus processable.

4. Desensitization and reprocessing
   The processing of the trauma network takes place using bilateral stimulation (usually eye movement). If a stress level (SUD) of 0 is reached, this phase is completed.
5. Anchoring of the target thought (positive cognition)
6. Body test
   If available, residues of a "body memory" are processed here.
7. Conclusion
8. Evaluation

Meanwhile, the efficacy of EMDR is not only known for PTSD, but also for a number of other diseases. Among other things, EMDR is also used to treat depression, anxiety / panic disorders, chronic pain and addiction.

6.5.2 Narrative Exposure Therapy (NET)

The Narrative Expositions-Therapie (NET) was developed by Maggie Schauer, Frank Neuner and Thomas Elbert at the University of Konstanz. It is originally intended for the treatment of severely and multiply traumatized people. NET was designed as a short-term therapy.

The aim of the therapy is to make the traumatic memory become part of the functioning autobiographical memory.

In order to achieve this, the individual's life story is worked out in the therapy session. During this work, the therapist pays attention to the so-called "hot spots", that is, those memories of the trauma that are not yet sufficiently integrated into the autobiographical memory. At this point, the progress of the narration of the affected person is slowed down and one focuses on the "hot spot". These "hot spots" should be told and re-experienced by the affected persons as intensively and in all qualities (thoughts, feelings, behavior, bodily experience) as possible. At the same time, the focus is on the feelings that arise in the situation of narration. At the end of the treatment, the feelings of "there and then" should be clearly distinguished from the feelings of "here and now".

6.5.3 PITT and Observer Technique

Luise Reddemann began in the 1980s, from a psychodynamic understanding, the Psychodynamic-Imaginary Trauma-Therapy (PITT) to develop. Meanwhile, the PITT is a therapy that is used in German-speaking countries for many sufferers of complex PTSD. The PITT is not a pure therapy for exposure therapy, but includes all phases of trauma therapy.

Basic principles of PITT are the following:
1. Release of the affected from external stress, e.g. by a hospital stay
2. The analytic abstinence rule is modified, which leads to the therapist being more active in the relationship
3. Activation of positive emotions
4. Establishment of strategies for self-soothing
5. Psychoeducation
6. Strengthening of resources and appreciation of defense mechanisms
7. Integration of imagination, mindfulness and cognitive restructuring
8. Avoidance of interpretation and confrontation
9. Promotion of progression
10. Working with personality aspects (so-called ego-states)

PITT has a special technique called the "inner stage". This imaginary space provides room for the visual representation of aspects, such as the "inner child". On this inner stage, interactions between different parts can take place under therapeutic supervision. Here, the "inner stage" is to be understood as a correspondence to the internalized object relationships.

The "inner child work" became particularly well-known, which is very similar to the work on the "inner stage". In this case, the ego-state is focused on, which represents the injured inner child. Then contact is made with this part. One tries to communicate imaginatively with this ego-state, whether verbally or non-verbally. In addition, the thoughts, feelings, body sensations and needs of this inner child find their place. To some extent, this child is also taken care of or brought to a safe place.

- **The Observer Technique**

A similar exercise (screen technique), as the observer technique, was already mentioned above under "dealing with flashbacks". This technique is also used as a confrontation technique in combination with PITT.

Before this technique is used to confront a memory, the client is given a thorough explanation of the procedure. The client is asked to imagine a large screen or canvas in front of them, against a real wall, in order to practice the technique. They should then pictorially imagine a pleasant memory from their life, experienced from a third person perspective. It is important that the client remains an observer of what is being projected. The therapist and client will then observe what is being projected together. The client should then imagine that they have a remote control for this projection. With this remote control, they can now control the projected memory. The image can be changed from color to black and white. The image can be paused, rewound, or fast forwarded. The sound can be turned up or the voices and noises can be distorted. The client should also practice changing the distance from the image or film. The observer decides how much contact they want with the image. Ultimately, the client should practice being able to turn the screen off, or draw a curtain in front of the canvas. This practice should create a distance that is necessary when confronted with the traumatic memory.

If the observer technique has been practiced sufficiently and all other conditions for the confrontation are met and there is enough stability, then the trauma can be processed. The client does not project a subjectively pleasant memory, but the traumatic one. As with the pleasant memory, the client should take on a third person perspective. This allows the contact with the trauma to be self-regulated and portioned. The affected person works through the traumatic memory with therapeutic accompaniment and should gradually gain control over the memories. In addition, the emotions that arise can be named and distinguished. At the end of each confrontation session, there should be a phase of self-calming and self-comfort. Before the session ends, it should be clarified exactly what support is now necessary and how it can be obtained.

6.5.4 IRRT

> **IRRT**
>
> IRRT stands for Imagery Rescripting and Reprocessing Therapy and was developed in the 1990s by psychologist Prof. Mervin Smucker to treat PTSD.

An IRRT confrontation session takes place in the imagination, if possible with closed eyes.

In the first phase, the client is asked to recall the traumatic experience in the imagination (i.e. on the inner stage) and then to tell the scene from beginning to end in the present tense, i.e. as if the scene were happening now.

In the second phase, the same scene is run through again imaginatively, but now an imaginative change takes place: The client enters the inner stage in the present, current (adult) self and disempowers the perpetrator. This should also remain in the present tense and the disempowerment should not take place as a theoretical construct, but quite concretely on the imaginative level of action. After the disempowerment, the third phase follows.

This third phase is characterized by the fact that the current self takes care of the former, injured (childish) self on the inner stage and provides for it. The aim is to achieve self-soothing and self-comfort, sometimes also reconciliation with oneself.

IRRT sessions are usually recorded on an audio carrier so that the client can listen to them during the week until the next therapy session. It should be discussed in advance how, when and where this will take place. Through this repetition of the confrontation with what happened in the therapy session, the client notices how the level of stress decreases with each listening.

6.6 Medication

Medications play only a subordinate role in the treatment of PTSD. There are only a few medications that have a direct effect on the core symptoms of PTSD. For the group of selective serotonin reuptake inhibitors (SSRIs), actually an antidepressant, an efficacy on the PTSD-specific symptoms is described. For this reason, these medications are also the first choice. The best evidence is for the efficacy of paroxetine and sertraline. In Germany, only paroxetine is approved for the treatment of PTSD. Other antidepressants, such as NSRIs and tricyclic antidepressants, should be used if treatment with an SSRI is not sufficient.

Benzodiazepines are often prescribed, especially for the treatment of overexcitement. On the one hand, these anxiolytics have an addictive potential, that is, they can lead to addiction with longer use, on the other hand, studies have shown that taking them, especially very shortly after the trauma, leads to an increased rate of PTSD. For this reason, treatment with benzodiazepines should be carried out carefully, indicated well and only after extensive counseling.

Other medications may be used for an additional comorbid disorder. For example, if there is a comorbid depression, a sensible antidepressant medication should be initiated. Medication should be in the hands of an experienced psychiatrist.

Overview of drugs that can be used in the treatment of PTSD:

Medication in the Treatment of PTSD
- Selective serotonin reuptake inhibitors (Selective Serotonin-Reuptake-Inhibitors = SSRI):
  - Drug of first choice!
  - Effectiveness also in PTSD-specific symptoms
  - Effectiveness best documented for paroxetine and sertraline
  - in Germany is only paroxetine approved
- Tricyclic antidepressants:
  - if SSRI are not enough
- Benzodiazepines:
  - Effect against symptoms of overexcitement
  - Caution due to potential for dependency
  - No administration shortly after trauma

References

AWMF-S3-Leitlinien Posttraumatische Belastungsstörung. (2001). AWMF-Registrierungsnummer 051–010.

Foa, E. B., Hembree, E. A., & Rothbaum, B. O. (2007). *Prolonged exposure therapy for PTSD: Emotional processing of traumatic experiences*. Oxford University Press.

Kanfer, F. H., Reinecker, H., & Schmelzer, D. (2006). *Selbstmanagementtherapie. Ein Lehrbuch für die klinische Praxis* (4th ed.). Springer.

Kubany, E. S. (1997). Thinking errors, faulty conclusions, and cognitive therapy for trauma-related guilt. *Nathinal Center for Post-Traumatic Stress Disorder Clinical Quarterly, 8*, 6–8.

Matten, S. J., & Pausch, M. J. (2017). *Angst- uns Panikstörungen im Beruf*. Kohlhammer.

Reddemann, L. (2007). *Imagination als heilsame Kraft. Zur Behandlung von Traumafolgen mit resourcenorientierten Verfahren* (13th ed.). Klett-Cotta.

Reddemann, L., Hofmann, A., & Gast, U. (Eds.) (2007). *Psychotherapie der dissoziativen Störungen* (2nd ed.). Georg Thieme.

Segal, Z. V., Williams, J. M. G., & Teasdale, J. D. (2008). *Die achtsamkeitsbasierte kognitive Therapie der Depression. Ein neuer Ansatz zur Rückfallprävention*. Dgvt-Verlag.

Shapiro, F. (2013). *Eye movement desensitization and reprocessing (EMDR) therapy: Basic principles, protocols, and procedures* (1st ED.). Guilford Publication; 1995, 2001 Deutsch: EMDR – Grundlagen und Praxis. 2. überarb. Aufl. Paderborn: Junfermann

Shapiro, F. (1991). Eye movement desensitization and reprocessing: A cautionary note. *The Behavior Therapist, 14*, 188.

How the Social Environment of Those Affected by Trauma and PTSD Deals with the Topic

The social environment of a person in the public eye, such as a manager, politician or actor, can in addition to direct professional and private contacts, such as family and friends, under certain circumstances also the whole society be in which the affected person moves. Thus, both the question "how does society deal with the issue of psychological trauma?" and the question "how does the close personal environment feel about it?" must be asked. As a result, the actually relevant question is asked: "What does this mean for the affected person?"

A definition "of society" is hardly possible, because it is too diverse and can be internationally different. But precisely with such questions and at this level there is a certain common view in Western Europe and North America. This is often not reflected, one tends to ignore the topics of trauma and fear and is rather negative towards them. In doubt, an affected person is interpreted as a weakness. Not surprisingly, it is a challenge for the authors to find partners for a foreword to this publication from public, politics and business. Hardly anyone dares to express themselves generally and certainly not personally in such a context and thus to position themselves. Because this could possibly be used negatively against the person concerned and such an attack surface is not even offered. Liberalism and solidarity therefore end quickly as soon as one is directly or indirectly affected, because then it is a matter of putting theoretical positions into practice. The concern described in this book, as an affected person of trauma or PTSD, to expect negative consequences in the event of careless communication, is therefore not unfounded. But as already mentioned, this should not lead to not seeking professional help. If society is already problematic with this overall topic, the immediate environment is all the more important.

Whether it's a colleague, friend or family member, whether for purely economic or personal reasons, an appropriate approach to this topic is of great importance and has significant meaning for the person concerned. Whether society is solidary with a person concerned or rejects and evaluates him negatively, rarely has anything to do with actual reasons and is subject to many partly uncontrollable factors. In doubt, a negative pressure must be expected, which in addition to the existing problem acts negatively and aggravatingly on the person concerned. This happens under certain circumstances completely independent of actual reasons and contexts of the traumatic background. The person concerned should not and cannot use his energies for this possible fight against society, that is a question of the sensible use of his own and thus of course limited resources. In the best case, this can be given to experienced press spokespersons or other professional and experienced service providers. The focus of the person concerned must remain on himself and the problem solving. The person concerned must also not be deterred by this possible negative handling of the society with the topic and the resulting consequences from becoming active. And if only in a very protected environment, for example in cooperation with a personal coach.

If it is involved, the personal environment of a person concerned therefore has the important task of stabilizing and supporting this person, perhaps also of providing shielding. Every person concerned is quite capable of coping without this support and of recovering, but this obviously has a positive and accelerated effect. The first and most important thing is to gain a comprehensive understanding of the situation and the context, making sure that the interests of the person concerned and not one's own interests and fears are really in focus. A possibly negative and therefore possibly additional burden on the person concerned can be greatly relativized in its importance. Here, too, the person concerned has a very important role to play: Not every comment in social networks, TV, press or other public must be taken seriously and thought through. But of course this is often difficult. Neither complete avoidance of communication and interaction nor the claim to be able to control everything is realistically acceptable. There is also rarely a clear right or wrong. The person concerned is affected and has enough other worries and needs his energy elsewhere. A positive approach of the social environment of a person concerned to the topic therefore has a very important meaning for the person concerned, who needs a safe space to move and communicate. This also applies to people who are not necessarily dependent on it.

Disease Prevention and Primary/Secondary Traumatization

Contents

8.1 **Prevention** – 100

8.2 **Secondary Traumatization** – 101

References – 101

© The Author(s), under exclusive license to Springer Fachmedien Wiesbaden GmbH, part of Springer Nature 2022
M. J. Pausch and S. J. Matten, *Trauma and Trauma Consequence Disorder*,
https://doi.org/10.1007/978-3-658-38807-2_8

8.1 Prevention

The prevention of diseases has the goal of maintaining or improving the health of people. The most important strategy is that the triggers of diseases are reduced or even eliminated. There is a distinction between primary, secondary and tertiary prevention.

In primary prevention it is about preventing the onset of diseases. This can be achieved through education and information. This includes, for example, the information on the risks of alcohol consumption, which is intended to prevent alcohol consumption and thus no alcohol dependencies occur. Another example would be the information measures on nicotine consumption.

In the context of PTSD, these are primary prevention measures that prepare for a potential traumatic experience.

In the first step, it is about identifying groups of people who are at particularly high risk of being exposed to a traumatic situation. Such risk groups are, for example, employees of the police, the armed forces or the rescue service. These groups of people should be protected from PTSD by professional and structured measures. Possible strategies for primary prevention of PTSD are (O'Brien, 1998; Sorenson, 2002):

1. Detailed discussion of the potentially traumatic moments.
2. The affected persons should be informed in advance about the possible danger of a traumatic moment. These moments should be discussed with them and already subjected to a cognitive assessment in advance. In addition, there should be a good exchange between experienced and less experienced people.
3. Information and education about the physiology and psychology of traumatic situations and about the symptoms of PTSD and their treatment.
4. "Dry run" of these moments.
5. Situations that represent an extreme burden and thus particularly involve the danger of traumatization should be played through in training situations so that it is possible to become familiar with such situations without extreme stress.
6. Working out and practicing the behavior in such moments.
7. Behaviors in situations of extreme stress should be practiced over and over again, so that a kind of automation arises. This creates a feeling of security.
8. Identification, naming, conscious perception and learning of coping strategies (= coping strategies) as well as strategies for tension regulation and relaxation.
9. The existing coping and stress regulation mechanisms should be recognized, named and used consciously. In addition, other, not yet existing coping strategies and relaxation strategies should be learned.

As part of secondary prevention a disease is already present, usually in the early stages, and its progression should be stopped. This is done through early diagnosis and early treatment. Breast and colon cancer screening are examples of secondary prevention.

Tertiary prevention includes all measures that are intended to reduce the severity or spread of a disease. This also includes relapse prevention. An example of a tertiary-preventive measure is rehabilitation.

8.2 Secondary Traumatization

Secondary traumatization is when someone experiences symptoms of PTSD after hearing about a traumatic event from someone who experienced it. This person has never experienced a traumatic event themselves, but they develop PTSD because they are hearing about such moments from, for example, a psychotherapist. To a certain extent, the occurrence of symptoms of PTSD or PTSD-like symptoms after being confronted with the trauma of the actual victim is a normal reaction. People who are affected by such secondary traumatization are often those who deal with trauma victims as part of their job, such as psychotherapists, police officers, and clergy.

To prevent secondary PTSD, the following measures are recommended:
1. Self-observation and self-verbalization
   The emotional, cognitive, and physical reactions during and after working with people with PTSD should be observed and named exactly. It should be noted whether these reactions have anything to do with the descriptions and reactions of the other person.
   The ability to recognize when working with people with PTSD whether one's own reaction has anything to do with the other person or not should be gained through good and sound self-experience (e.g. as part of psychotherapist training).
2. Self-care/self-protection
   It is of great importance in the direct work with the people affected by PTSD as well as afterwards that attention is paid to self-care/-protection. There should always be a possibility to distance oneself from the other person's story. If, during the work with people with PTSD, the feeling arises of being overwhelmed, it is legitimate and necessary to say "stop" early. What applies to people with PTSD must also apply to the listener. Here one should always be aware of one's function as a role model. By saying "stop", people with PTSD can learn that it is quite all right and even good to pay attention to self-protection and self-care early on.
3. Organization of work/supervision/intervision
   Wherever possible, contacts with PTSD sufferers should be arranged in such a way that there is a moment of peace before and after. Perhaps a specific distancing or relaxation exercise should also be carried out when the PTSD sufferer has left.
   In addition, regular supervision and intervision should take place. The exchange with colleagues and the re-examination of the work with PTSD sufferers by a supervisor provide relief and space for one's own person.
4. Leisure activities
   Working with PTSD sufferers can be beautiful, satisfying and fulfilling, but it is always stressful and requires energy. Attention should be paid to a conscious balance. Where are your own resources? How is your own resilience strengthened?

References

O'Brien, S. L. (Ed.). (1998). *Traumatic events and mental health*. University Press.
Sorenson, S. B. (2002). Preventing traumatic stress: Public health approaches. *Journal of Traumatic Stress*, *15*, 3–7.

Trauma and PTSD in Film and Literature

Contents

9.1   Movies with the Theme of Trauma and PTSD – 104

9.2   Literary Works with the Theme of Trauma and PTSD – 106

© The Author(s), under exclusive license to Springer Fachmedien Wiesbaden GmbH, part of Springer Nature 2022
M. J. Pausch and S. J. Matten, *Trauma and Trauma Consequence Disorder*,
https://doi.org/10.1007/978-3-658-38807-2_9

Traumas, trauma-related disorders and PTSD in particular are often portrayed in movies and books. Most of the time, the trauma-related disorder or PTSD is not mentioned directly, but only described in terms of symptoms. Influenced by the experiences of the Vietnam War, especially in the 1970s and 1980s, movies were made that had PTSD as their subject matter. These movies deal with the individual biographies of Vietnam War veterans. The symptoms, the suffering, but also the difficulties in coping with everyday life after the war are the central themes of the movies. But even before and after the Vietnam War, filmmakers, screenwriters, writers and other artists dealt with the topic of traumatization, trauma-related disorder and PTSD. Now follows a small selection of movies and literary works in which a traumatization or PTSD plays an important role.

9.1 Movies with the Theme of Trauma and PTSD

- "Born on July 4th"

> Original title: "Born on the Fourth of July"
>
> Year of publication: 1989
>
> Director: Oliver Stone, Ron Kovic
>
> Screenplay: Oliver Stone
>
> Camera: Robert Richardson
>
> Actor: Tom Cruise (Ron Kovic)

Plot of the Film

In 1989, Oliver Stone directed the film "Born on the 4th of July". The film is based on the autobiography of Vietnam veteran Ron Kovic. Kovic was a Marine in the Vietnam War and was injured as a soldier in Vietnam, which led to him being paralyzed from the chest down. After returning from the Vietnam War, he became active in the anti-war movement. Tom Cruise plays the role of Ron Kovic. The film shows how the protagonist struggles with his physical and psychological consequences after returning from the war. The symptoms of PTSD are shown as well as the sometimes self-destructive attempts to deal with them. In addition, Kovic's development into a peace activist is shown. In 1990, Oliver Stone won an Oscar for his direction of "Born on the 4th of July" in the category of best director.

- "Rambo"

> Original title: "First Blood"
>
> Year of publication: 1982
>
> Director: Ted Kotcheff
>
> Screenplay: Michael Kozoll, William Sackheim, Sylvester Stallone
>
> Camera: Andrew Laszlo
>
> Actors: Sylvester Stallone (John J. Rambo), Richard Crenna (Col. Samuel Trautman), Brian Dennehy (Sheriff Will Teasle).

9.1 · Movies with the Theme of Trauma and PTSD

▪▪ Plot of the Film

Another film that deals with a Vietnam veteran as the protagonist is "Rambo". The film by Ted Kotcheff from the year 1982 is based on the novel "First Blood" by David Morrell. The main role of the war veteran John Rambo was played by Sylvester Stallone. The film, which falls into the category of action film, shows not only the individual difficulties of the protagonist but also the difficulties of the US American society with war returnees. Through a re-traumatization, "the fight for survival" takes place in John Rambo. In him, those behaviors and experiences become active again that he had to acquire in the Vietnam War in order to survive.

▪ Copykill

> Original title: "Copycat"
>
> Year of publication: 1995
>
> Director: Jon Amiel
>
> Screenplay: Ann Biderman, David Madsen
>
> Camera: László Kovács
>
> Actors: Sigourney Weaver (Helen Hudson), Holly Hunter (M. J. Monahan).

▪▪ Plot of the Film

Copykill is a US-American thriller from the year 1995 in which Sigourney Weaver plays the main role, a psychologist named Helen Hudson. As a psychologist, she worked as a profiler and specialized in serial killers. After an attempted murder on her by a serial killer, she suffers from a massive agoraphobia and takes pills and alcohol to calm down. After more than a year, she is contacted by a policewoman who hopes for help in the investigation of a serial murder. Helen Hudson, who has not left her apartment since the attempted murder and only communicates with the world via the Internet, is reminded of her own story by this request. The symptoms of post-traumatic stress disorder and the attempts to deal with them are shown, as well as the existential threat that arises when approaching one's own traumatic memories.

▪ Mystic River

> Original title: "Mystic River"
>
> Year of publication: 2003
>
> Director: Clint Eastwood
>
> Screenplay: Brian Helgeland
>
> Camera: Tom Stern
>
> Actors: Sean Penn (Jimmy Markum), Tim Robbins (Dave Boyle), Kevin Bacon (Sean Devine), Laurence Fishburne (Sgt. Whitey Powers).

■ ■ Plot of the Film

Mystic River is a film adaptation of the novel of the same name by Dennis Lehane from 2003. Clint Eastwood directed it. The film is about the three friends Jimmy Markum (played by Sean Penn), Dave Boyle (Tim Robbins) and Sean Devine (Kevin Bacon). At the age of about 11, Dave Boyle is abused and raped for 4 days until he finally manages to escape. 25 years later, the three friends meet again. Jimmy is now a former criminal who runs a small supermarket, and Sean has become a police officer. After a murder, which Sean investigates, Dave becomes the main suspect. Dave is again brought into contact with his own tragic story by what happens in the here and now. He is still not able to talk about what happened to him as a child.

9.2 Literary Works with the Theme of Trauma and PTSD

- "Macbeth"

> Original title: "The Tragedy of Macbeth"
>
> Original language: English
>
> Author: William Shakespeare
>
> Year of publication: 1623

■ ■ Action of the Work

William Shakespeare's tragedy "Macbeth" from the year 1606 is probably one of the most famous works of the poet. In it he describes how Macbeth becomes king of Scotland and then develops into a tyrant. Macbeth himself becomes king of Scotland through the murder of the king of Scotland carried out with his wife. Both Macbeth himself and his wife Lady Macbeth have repeated hallucinations, which can be seen as intrusions. Lady Macbeth suffers from sleep disorders, tormenting feelings of guilt and has the illusion in one scene (as part of an intrusion, since she actually had blood on her hands at the time of the murder) that there is still blood on her hands and she can not wash it off. In the end, she increasingly despair and finally takes her own life.

- "The Head of the Medusa" in Ovid's Metamorphoses

> Original title: "Metamorphoseon libri"
>
> Original language: Latin
>
> Author: Ovid
>
> Year of composition: 8 AD

■ ■ Plot of the Work

The Roman poet Ovid tells the story of the transformation and beheading of Medusa in the 4th book of the Metamorphoses. The story stands for abuse and the confrontation with it.

9.2 · Literary Works with the Theme of Trauma and PTSD

The Greek god of the sea, Poseidon, fell in love with the beautiful Medusa, a mortal daughter of Phorkys and Keto. Poseidon appears to Medusa in the form of a horse and "dishonors" her in the temple of Athena on the Acropolis of Athens. Medusa becomes pregnant with Poseidon. Athena turns Medusa—as punishment for this act—into a horrible creature with a long tongue, the tusks of a boar, bronze hands, golden wings and snake hair. At the sight of Medusa, everyone froze and turned to stone. Poseidon went unpunished. So there was a punishment of the victim of the abuse, while the perpetrator went unpunished.

Perseus finally sets out on the long journey to find Medusa and cut off her head. For this he receives a shiny bronze shield from Athena, a diamond sickle from Hermes and a cap, winged shoes and a sack from the nymphs. When he now finds Medusa, he only sees her reflection in the shiny shield and strikes her head with the sickle. From Medusa's body arise the giant Chrysaor and the winged horse Pegasus. It is said that coral formed from the drops of blood that spurted when her head was cut off.

In the language of trauma therapy, the long journey can be seen as the process of therapy itself. In order to deal with the horror of memory (here in the form of the head of Medusa with her snake hair and the petrification at her sight), the traveler needs "tools": a cap as a metaphor for the distancing techniques in flashbacks in trauma therapy, a "safe place" to which one can come with winged shoes, and a "vault" (sack for the head of Medusa) in order to be able to safely store the horror. The shield represents the view of what happened from a distance. By dealing with the horror of the deed, that is, the head of Medusa, it is possible to achieve a new strength, symbolized by the giant Chrysaor, and a creativity and spontaneity, symbolized by the horse Pegasus.

Future Prospects, Manage Business and Everyday Life

Contents

10.1 What Can I Do? – 110

10.2 Understanding as the First Step to a Solution – 111

© The Author(s), under exclusive license to Springer Fachmedien Wiesbaden GmbH, part of Springer Nature 2022
M. J. Pausch and S. J. Matten, *Trauma and Trauma Consequence Disorder*,
https://doi.org/10.1007/978-3-658-38807-2_10

Even if it often seems extremely unlikely from the perspective of those affected: Yes, it is possible to overcome PTSD and heal completely—no matter how far advanced. This is definitely a positive future perspective that can often not be seen so easily by the person affected for well understandable reasons. And no, this is not easy to achieve. In the rarest of cases, this succeeds by itself, neither by closing one's eyes nor by waiting it out. Active action, focus and targeted use of inner resources are necessary.

Business and everyday life cannot simply continue as before. But if you change and adapt them to your new needs, you can master both well and successfully. A simple "carry on!" usually leads to a worsening of the situation on all levels. A radical acceptance of the new situation is a prerequisite for a successful restructuring and the creation of a new foundation. Whether one wants to return to old patterns at all after a successful processing and perhaps even overcoming of a trauma or PTSD is another question that arises later.

10.1 What Can I Do?

First of all, take small steps. You don't have to decide and organize everything immediately. Assume that you are ill and need healing. And that this is not as short-term feasible or perhaps even ignorable as with a cold. Organize your environment anew and adapted to your needs. Do this in such a way that you have personal and time-out spaces left. Consider whether external support might be helpful in your case. If so: What form is suitable for you? If you need support, get it. Try to avoid short-term, simple solutions and focus on sustainability. The primary goal should be to become completely healthy. Secondarily, your family and, if applicable, your career. Thirdly, your profession in general as well as your social environment. Set priorities, create your very own emergency plan. If you need professional support, don't hesitate. Now you are creating basics. Without health, all other factors are meaningless and can't build on anything. Simply assuming "it will work out" can quickly become overwhelming and make the situation much worse. The affected person is hardly able to make an objective assessment of the situation at this point, as too many unknown factors come into play and he cannot fall back on experience values. This is even the case if the person affected should manage to take a completely independent, external view of the situation. But even this is actually hardly possible. Accept what has happened and try to determine where you stand—completely independent of possible reasons why it happened. Define your status quo with a view to the future. If you find support helpful, organize it. Make your decisions based on this result. This is a typical, familiar approach; you would do the same as a manager in a crisis situation. All points can be approached and resolved purely rationally. An possibly overwhelming emotional commitment is not necessary. The goal should be to create basics and set switches so that you can take a path that could lead to your recovery. Everything else may also be important and worth considering, but it can only be secondary to this.

10.2 Understanding as the First Step to a Solution

"Understanding"—yes, but what exactly? Understanding the new situation? But how is it actually? And according to which parameters can this be quantitatively and qualitatively measurable? Or is this classification simply "by feeling" possible, so to speak an estimate?

It is certainly a mixture of everything and neither a purely rational nor a purely emotional approach can give a correct overall picture. In order to be able to make any meaningful assessment at all, a first understanding of what has happened and the resulting consequences is necessary. Especially people in management and public are this—intellectually seen—easier possible, but practically seen these people often do not see "the forest in front of the trees" and trust their intuitions too little. Because especially these have become confused and therefore difficult to assess.

Understanding the reasons and connections facilitates the dealing with the new situation. A high degree of ability to introspection can be helpful at this point, but is not absolutely necessary. The will, together with the active implementation of an as comprehensive understanding as possible, is sufficient and a first important step. Based on this, initial decisions, such as the involvement of external, possibly professional support, can be made.

Supplementary Information

Recommended Reading – 114

Index – 115

© The Editor(s) (if applicable) and The Author(s), under exclusive license to Springer Fachmedien Wiesbaden GmbH, part of Springer Nature 2022
M. J. Pausch and S. J. Matten, *Trauma and Trauma Consequence Disorder*,
https://doi.org/10.1007/978-3-658-38807-2

Recommended Reading

Butollo, W., & Hagl, M. (2003). *Trauma, Selbst und Therapie. Konzepte und Kontroversen in der Psychotraumatologie*. Huber.

Hayes, S. C., & Smith, S. (2007). In *Abstand zur inneren Wortmaschine. Ein Selbsthilfe- und Therapiebegleitbuch auf der*

Huber, M. (2006). *The ways of trauma treatment. Trauma and trauma treatment part 2* (3rd ed.). Junfermann.

Huber, M. (2007). *Trauma and its consequences. Trauma and trauma treatment. Part 1* (3rd ed.). Junfermann.

Kabat-Zinn, J. (2009). *Gesund durch Meditation. Das große Buch der Selbstheilung*. Fischer Taschenbuch.

Linehan, M. (1996). *Dialectical-behavioral therapy of borderline personality disorder*. CIP-Medien.

Maercker, A. (2013). *Posttraumatic stress disorder*. Springer.

Matten, S. J., & Pausch, M. J. (2017). *Angst- uns Panikstbergtungsstapie*. Kohlhammer.

Reddemann, L. (2007). *Imagination als heilsame Kraft. Zur Behandlung von Traumafolgen mit resourcenorientierten Verfahren* (13th ed.). Klett-Cotta.

Sachsse, U. (Ed.). (2004). *Traumazentrierte Psychotherapie. Theorie, Klinik und Praxis*. Schattauer.

Sasse, U. (2004). *Traumazentrierte Psychotherapie. Theorie, Klinik und Praxis*. Schattauer.

Schmucker, M., & Köster, R. (2015). *Praxishandbuch IRRT Imagery Rescripting & Reprocessing Therapy bei Traumafolgestr/43130" esourcenorientierten Verfahr*. Klett-Cotta.

Shapiro, F. (2013a). *EMDR processing therapy for trauma-related disorders: A resource-oriented approach*. Junfermann.

van der Hart, O., Nijenhuis, R. S. E., Steele, K., & Kierdorf, T, (2008). *The haunted self: Structural dissociation and the treatment of chronic traumatization*. Junfermann.

Index

3-2-1-exercise 88
100-minus-7-Übung 63

A

A1 criterion 9
Accidental traumas 5
Active communication 57
Acute stress reaction 7
Addiction 81
– comorbidity 47
Adjustment disorder 7
Affected 2, 4–6, 8, 10, 11, 14–16, 18–23, 26, 28, 30, 31, 33, 34, 36, 37, 40–42, 46–48, 50, 54–57, 61, 62, 64, 65, 67, 72–77, 79–85, 88–93, 96, 97, 100, 101, 110
Agoraphobia 40
Alcohol dependence 45
American Psychiatric Association 5
Amygdala 31
ANP (atrial natriuretic peptide) 20
Anxiety 5, 7–10, 26, 28, 40, 41, 43, 45, 48, 54, 66, 78, 85, 91
Anxiety disorder 40
– comorbidity 43, 45, 50, 85
– generalized 42
Anxiety management 66, 78
Anxiety state 28
Attachment system 17
Autogenic training 70
Avoidance 7–9, 28, 29, 32–35, 39–42, 45, 65, 66, 78, 97
Avoidance behavior 28, 33
– reduction 66

B

Blame 56
Body scan meditation 87
Book 2, 8, 12, 31, 34, 50, 96, 104, 106
Breathing exercise 68
Broca Language Center 17
Brooding 77
Business 14, 15, 30, 33, 35, 46, 48, 49, 55, 73, 96, 110

C

Case example 18, 30, 32, 39, 49
Challenge 2, 15, 89, 96
Cognitive behavioral therapy 84
Cognitive bias 56
Cognitive processing therapy 84
Cognitive trap 74, 76
Comorbidity 39
Complex PTSD 8, 34
Complex trauma disorder 8
Confrontation 5, 23, 29, 81, 83, 84, 88, 89, 92, 93, 106
Coping mechanism 20
Core symptom 8
Cortex 16
Counter stimuli (Skill) 62
Crisis management 57

D

Danger 14
Debriefing 23
– phases 23
Definition 4
Dell 37
Dependence disorder 45
– comorbidity 39
Depression 44
– comorbidity 45
DESNOS 8
Detoxification treatment 47
Diagnostic criteria
– DIS 37
DIS (dissociative identity disorder) 36
– characteristics 37
Dissociation 16, 17, 19, 36, 72
– relatives 74
Dissociation chain 72
Dissociative identity structure 39
Distancing technique 88
DSM 5
DSM-5 9

E

Early intervention 21, 22
Ego-State 36
EMDR (Eye Movement Desensitization and Reprocessing) 90
Emergency plan 110
Emergency psychology 21
Emotion 15
Emotion research 14
EP (evoked potentials) 20
Escape 17
Example 25, 45
Example case 33, 34, 43, 47, 50
Existential threat 16
Extremsituation 16

F

Fear 78
Feeling 14
Fight 16, 17
Film 18, 29, 61, 65, 92
Flash-back 32, 62
Flash-back-chain 62
Flight 16

G

Generalized anxiety disorder 42
Guilt 8, 9, 14, 34, 44, 47, 50, 106

H

Herausforderung 15
High-risk behavior 50
High-risk hypothesis 46
Hippocampus 17
Hopelessness 4
How Skills 86
Hyperarousal 28, 32, 33

I

ICD-10 7
– DIS 37
– F43.1 7
Imagery Rescripting and Reprocessing Therapy (IRRT) 84, 93
Imagination exercise 64, 67–69, 86
Inner safe place 68, 89

Intentional traumas 5
Introspection 111
Intrusion 28, 30, 32, 33, 61
IRRT (imagery rescripting and reprocessing therapy) 84, 93

L

Late-onset-PTSD 21

M

Manager 56
Man-made-disaster 5
Medication 28, 44, 47, 50, 93, 94
Mindfulness 85
Mood 15
Movie 104

N

NET 91
Nightmare 32
Numbness 20

O

Obesity
– comorbidity 49
Overweight
– comorbidity 49

P

Pain 6, 18, 20, 24, 30, 36, 40, 50, 51
Panic disorder 41
Perpetrator introject 50
Phobia
– social 41
– specific 42
PITT (psychodynamic-imaginative trauma therapy) 84, 91
Post-Traumatic Stress Disorder 6–8
Powernapping 65
Pressure of suffering 15
Prevention 100
– primary 100

– secondary 100, 101
– tertiary 100
Problem solving 56, 96
Prodromi 61
Progressive muscle relaxation 67, 71
Prolonged exposure 84
Psychodynamic-Imaginative Trauma Therapy (PITT) 84, 91
Psychoeducation 22
Psychomotor agitation 20
Psychotherapy phases 83
PTSD (post-traumatic stress disorder) 2, 6–12, 14, 21–23, 25, 26, 34, 39, 40, 43, 45–48, 50, 56, 57, 89, 91–94, 96, 100, 101, 104, 110

R

Radical acceptance 87
Railway spine syndrome 11
Rape
– frequency 10
Reality control 63
Relationship traumatization 5
Reorientation 81, 83, 89
Resilience 23
Resistance 23
Resource 81
Resource diagram 82
Risk factor 6, 12, 22, 25

S

Safe exercise 64
Screen exercise 64
Screen technique 92
Secondary traumatization 101
Self-confidence 24
Self-help group 46, 47, 81
Self-injurious behavior 50
Self-medication hypothesis 45
Sensitivity hypothesis 46
Severity 4
Skill 73
Sleep disorder 31, 80
Social environment 96
Social network 24, 54
Social phobia 41
Society 96

Specific phobia 42
Splitting 19
Stabilization 85
Strength 54
Substance abuse counselor 40, 46
Suddenness 4
Suffering 15, 21, 31, 32, 34, 36–38, 66, 72, 75, 80, 86, 87, 104
Suicidal thoughts 50
Survival 16
Survivor syndrome 11
Symptom 54

T

Taste intrusion 30, 62
Therapeutic goal 23
Therapy goal 82
Thought circles 77
Threat
– existential 16
Trauma disorder 6
Trauma-focused cognitive behavioral therapy 84
Trauma network 18
Traumatic pincer 16
Traumatic vice 19
Traumatization
– secondary 101
– severe 34
Treatment options 61
Trigger 72
Type-II-Traumata 5
Type-I-Traumata 5

V

Violent crime
– frequency 10

W

Walking meditation 87
War tremblers 11
Weakness 54
What Skills 86
Wise mind 86
Withdrawal treatment 38, 46, 47, 81, 85
Worry book 77

GPSR Compliance

The European Union's (EU) General Product Safety Regulation (GPSR) is a set of rules that requires consumer products to be safe and our obligations to ensure this.

If you have any concerns about our products, you can contact us on

ProductSafety@springernature.com

In case Publisher is established outside the EU, the EU authorized representative is:

Springer Nature Customer Service Center GmbH
Europaplatz 3
69115 Heidelberg, Germany

www.ingramcontent.com/pod-product-compliance
Ingram Content Group UK Ltd.
Pitfield, Milton Keynes, MK11 3LW, UK
UKHW050507040925
462575UK00015B/698